The Doctor's
QUICK WEIGHT LOSS
Diet

BY

Irwin Maxwell Stillman, M.D.,D-IM

AND

Samm Sinclair Baker

A DELL BOOK

With love to my wife Ruth
I.M.S.

Published by

DELL PUBLISHING CO., INC.
750 Third Avenue
New York, N.Y. 10017

First Dell printing—August 1968
Second Dell printing—September 1968
Third Dell printing—October 1968
Fourth Dell printing—October 1968
Fifth Dell printing—December 1968
Sixth Dell printing—January 1969
Seventh Dell printing—March 1969
Eighth Dell printing—April 1969
Ninth Dell printing—May 1969
Tenth Dell printing—May 1969
Eleventh Dell printing—May 1969
Twelfth Dell printing—July 1969
Thirteenth Dell printing—October 1969
Fourteenth Dell printing—November 1969
Fifteenth Dell printing—November 1969
Sixteenth Dell printing—December 1969
Seventeenth Dell printing—February 1970
Eighteenth Dell printing—April 1970
Nineteenth Dell printing—May 1970
Twentieth Dell printing—May 1970
Twenty-First Dell printing—November 1970
Twenty-Second Dell printing—March 1971
Twenty-Third Dell printing—April 1971
Twenty-Fourth Dell printing—June 1971
Twenty-Fifth Dell printing—July 1971
Twenty-Sixth Dell printing—September 1971
Twenty-Seventh Dell printing—November 1971
Twenty-Eighth Dell printing—December 1971
Twenty-Ninth Dell printing—February 1972
Thirtieth Dell printing–April 1972
Thirty-First Dell printing—May 1972

From The Doctor's Casebook:

Mrs. F.G. weighed 194 lbs. and was only 5'1". She had tried to reduce 14 different times without success. The Doctor's Quick Weight Loss Diet helped her lose 10 lbs. the first week. Within a year she was at 105 lbs., which she has maintained.

Mr. D.E., at age 32, was 243 lbs. instead of 153–170, the ideal weight, and he suffered from high blood pressure. The diet put him down to 183 lbs. in 14 weeks. He'll stabilize at about 165 lbs. His blood pressure has dropped and he feels like a new man.

Mrs. E.F. weighed 155 lbs. instead of her ideal weight of under 110 lbs. for her 5'2". In two months on the Doctor's Quick Weight Loss Diet she was down to 115 lbs.

During his fifty years of experience in the practice of medicine, Irwin Maxwell Stillman, M.D., has helped over 10,000 overweight men and women to reduce. A Diplomate in Internal Medicine, Dr. Stillman is presently a consultant in Internal Medicine at Coney Island Hospital, Brooklyn, New York. Formerly, he was an attending physician in Medicine at Coney Island Hospital, an attending physician in Medicine at Harbor Hospital, a clinical instructor of Medicine at Long Island College Hospital, a Fellow of the American College of Angiology, and a Fellow of the American Geriatric Society.

Contents

The Doctor's
QUICK WEIGHT LOSS
Diet

1. THE QUICK WEIGHT LOSS DIET SUCCEEDS WHERE OTHERS FAIL

The prime aim of this book is to *take that weight off you quickly*, and then to help you stay slim, healthy and attractive. Here you'll learn exactly how in clear, simple, *proved* ways never told to you before.

You can achieve your desired weight reduction, no matter how many times you may have failed up to now. That's because you'll be using the Quick Weight Loss Diet and other speedy, safe and effective reducing procedures I have developed in treating over 10,000 overweight men and women in more than 45 years of medical practice.

The necessary, workable instructions that have helped my patients are condensed for you on these pages. All essential details are included. Your special advantage is having the directions handy always for repeated reference and checking.

Once down to your ideal size and figure, you're not left to fight weight increase on your own. As my patients have done with triumphant success, you follow through with the Quick Loss and Stay Slim Eating Combination. You'll find it as easy and remarkably effective as they have. It can work wonderfully for you for the rest of your healthier, more vigorous life.

There are specific built-in reasons why the Quick Weight Loss Diet has succeeded with many hard-to-reduce women and men who had just about given up hope of ever being slim again. Here are the most important:

1. Much more of the body fat is burned off with the

Quick Weight Loss Diet than with most other diets, including the most rigorous and difficult. Eating this way you consume fewer calories each day; also your system burns up about 275 *more calories daily* than with a diet of the same total calorie intake that includes other foods.

2. You don't count calories on the Quick Weight Loss Diet, although calories *do* count. What happens is that you're taking in fewer calories daily without keeping track of them. As you eat, you find that your food consumption is self-limiting. You eat plenty but you don't "hunger" for more than will take off weight quickly.

3. You lose weight rapidly with the Quick Weight Loss Diet which alone is a great aid in continuing the diet.

4. It's a relatively easy reducing method to follow when you're dining out in restaurants. This has proved to be a crucial asset for busy overweight men and women among my patients. You are permitted just about as many helpful "coffee breaks" as you want, within the dieting method.

5. At intervals, as many of my patients do, you return to the Quick Weight Loss Diet if necessary for only a few days or a week to keep extra pounds from "creeping up" on you. The unique combination of intermittent Quick Loss and Stay Slim Eating, as given later in detail, will help you once and for all to take off poundage and then stay slim thereafter.

Only this dieting method helped me bring down my weight from 190 to 140 pounds quickly. I would have been dead years ago if I hadn't taken off that excess fat in a hurry. The same is true of many who have used this diet. This includes doctors and their wives and families, nurses, dieticians, life insurance experts, actors, models and others who came to me because they had failed to reduce successfully with either various fads and gimmicks or on "regular reducing diets."

In one case, a woman who had "tried everything"

without being able to reduce, dropped 25 pounds the first week on the Quick Weight Loss Diet, 67 pounds in 4 months. She is now on the highly effective Combination Plan of Stay Slim Eating and occasional Quick Loss dieting which you will learn to apply for yourself. She is maintaining her ideal weight, has improved her health and has achieved a lovely slim figure, to the amazement and delight of her family and friends.

Hers is the largest weight loss in one week of any patient on my records, but a long-range loss is typical. Neither she nor any other of my patients, not a single one, suffered ill effects from quick and dramatic weight losses. Every one of them enjoyed a new glow of healthy vigor and vitality compared to their previous state. And each undoubtedly added years of life—buoyant, healthful years.

It is most satisfying and encouraging to a dieter to see the weight on the scale drop rapidly and the fat "melt away," as happens with this method. One patient who lost 8½ pounds in her first week on the diet told me, "After failing on many diets, the big loss the first week has given me the confidence I needed. I was never able to lose so much before. Now I know I can lose weight and I'll stick with it until I reach my goal of a youthful figure that will make people take notice."

You too will be so delighted and impressed by seeing the decided drop in weight when you step on the scale each morning, that you'll keep dieting another day, then another and another. Dieting "just one more day" is a key to success in losing weight. The aphorism applies that "nothing succeeds like success."

It's an unfortunate fact of the usually recommended slow "balanced dieting" that when a person sees his weight dropping only a pound or so a week, he invariably says, "What's the use of even trying? I'll never make it." And he goes back to stuffing himself again. But my records show that my considerably overweight patients averaged a loss of 6 to 7 pounds in the first

3 days on the Quick Weight Loss Diet, almost as dramatic as the loss on a fasting diet. Such impressive evidence that it worked, seeing results on the scale with their own eyes, kept them on the simple, plentiful, satisfying diet.

This method will take off excess weight for 95 out of every 100 persons. If you're one of the normal 95%, and you follow this diet and still don't lose weight rapidly but keep on gaining weight, *then you're lying to yourself and to others.*

It's a generally accepted estimate that only 5 out of every 100 persons have some metabolic disorder which keeps them from losing weight even on a rigid reducing schedule, only 5 percent of the entire population. If you're one of those rare 1-in-20 individuals, your doctor undoubtedly told you so on your last examination. If you have no such complicating physical disorder, this method will take off your excess weight; just follow the brief, uncomplicated instructions.

The situation that is overwhelmingly true of most overweight people is that you're kidding yourself if you think that some mysterious ailment would prevent you from reducing on this or any other diet. As a doctor advised a fat patient, "The tests show that your thyroid is normal, your problem is an overactive fork."

The Combination Plan solves another problem voiced by most dieters: "Sure, a stringent diet will take off weight for a little while, but then it comes right back. Whatever I lose, I'll gain back again—and more!" As a result of this prevalent conviction, you may have been so sure in the past that you couldn't succeed that you don't even start any more. But regaining lost weight need not happen, as thousands of my patients can tell you.

Using the Quick Weight Loss method combined with Stay Slim Eating, most of these men and women of all sizes, weights and ages have lost their dreadful excess poundage and have continued to maintain their ideal reduced weight according to my "Ideal Weight Table" (see Chapter 3).

This method acts to change your harmful overeating habits and to break the custom of gorging at meals and snacking continually on high calorie foods. In this way alone, by stopping vicious, harmful eating cycles, the diet rules help you to reduce and stay slim *after* the dieting period is past. Then the Combination Plan takes over to help you keep your weight down month after month and year after year.

Don't let the melancholy derogators of anything "new" discourage and deter you from starting the Quick Weight Loss Diet. Hundreds, thousands of overweight individuals have come to me with pleas like this: "Doctor, I've tried to cut down on my eating and calories on a 'balanced diet' but I just can't. I've failed dozens of times. Can you help me?"

According to those who advocate only "regular balanced dieting," I should answer, "I can't help you if you won't regulate your eating to limit yourself to smaller portions only of the foods on a 'balanced diet' list." But I know that most of them would fail again with such advice, like the all-too-typical fat lady in a cartoon who told a waiter, "I'll have a cup of bouillon, cottage cheese salad, melba toast, clear tea and, heaven help me, a banana split." Another moaned, "I went on one of those balanced diets for 4 weeks, but all I lost was 28 days."

The stark truth which must be faced by all, the medical profession and the public alike, is that most people who are overweight love to eat though they may deny it. When told to go on a reducing diet which usually consists primarily of eating smaller portions of a wide variety of foods, most of them just can't limit themselves. Even if they start, they can't stick to it. So they never really even get started.

YOUR GREATEST DANGER—
AND HOW TO OVERCOME IT

Back in 1959, Dr. Louis M. Orr, then president of the American Medical Association, was asked in a newspaper interview, "Do you consider cancer as the greatest threat we face?" He answered, "No. Cancer is the most dreaded disease in the United States. But the greatest danger to the health of the American people is obesity."

Now, years later, in spite of such warnings, tens of millions of Americans are overweight. They're not taking advantage of the quick weight loss techniques that work.

I'm constantly appalled by the ingrained conviction most fat people have, and too many wives, husbands, relatives and friends of overweights, that to change one's habits and eat "differently" is a harmful thing to do. Consider sensibly and calmly the illogic of this attitude: the way you've been eating has made you fat —*that's the way that's bad for you.*

Almost any change in the direction of consuming fewer calories must be a change for the better. And obviously the sooner you change, and usually the more drastically you change, the healthier you'll be, and the quicker.

Generalized advice which is usually fed to you, no matter how good it may be, seldom works for you. By following the specific dieting recommendations here you'll lose excess weight, continue on healthful stay slim eating, and never become a fatty again.

In my experience there's no question that quick-action dieting which alters radically and suddenly your ways of eating is the best way to reduce and enjoy the many health benefits that follow. Most overweights need the shock treatment of having their eating clearly defined by a specific diet plan which takes pounds off speedily and dramatically. That demonstrated proof of the promise is essential in order for most dieters to succeed. You then go on eagerly to lose the dangerous excess weight that it is urgent for you to take off for your health's sake.

With all its acknowledged benefits, being slim is not a cure-all in itself. Being at ideal weight is not a guarantee against all illness or of extra long life. But your chances of staying healthy or becoming healthier, of avoiding a heart attack and many other serious ailments, of living a longer, more vigorous lifetime, are increased enormously when you melt away layers and pockets of fat that burden your organs.

What's more, and this is of extreme importance in every facet of social and business life, you'll certainly look more attractive to yourself and to others. Most of my patients have accomplished all this safely and happily after other methods had failed for them, by using the quick loss dieting techniques detailed in this book.

I created the Quick Weight Loss Diet and the Combination Plan because my overweight patients needed this specific help. They had never succeeded in reducing on "regular balanced dieting."

I urge you to get started now on this diet. Every day that you delay and keep or increase that excess poundage is impairing your appearance and your health, and is endangering and shortening your life. Overweight is a kind of death for most everyone, slow for some, quicker for others.

When you've gotten down to your desired ideal weight and figure with this method, have a checkup by your doctor if you didn't consult him at the start. This will be valuable reassurance to you that not only didn't the dieting impair your health, but that you're in far better condition in every way.

Of course you'll know this already thanks to the wonderful difference in the way you feel and from the compliments you get on your improved appearance.

ANALYSIS OF THIRTY OVERWEIGHT PATIENTS

While writing this book I analyzed again the records of 30 of my most recent overweight patients. This special little study revealed interesting and promising facts for you:

First, it was remarkable how quickly and easily they all learned the Quick Weight Loss dieting technique and how uniformly it kept each one dieting and losing pounds (they dieted as individuals, not as a group).

Second, on the occasions when some of them slipped off the Quick Weight Loss Diet, they knew from experience that a return to it would take weight off rapidly. Each one went right back on the quick-reducing instructions.

Third, their records (and thousands of others) proved the fallacy of a too-prevalent viewpoint that a fast take-off of weight is linked inevitably with a fast put-on. This is not true. I have seen too many people struggle with slow-take-off diets, then slip and put on weight quickly—and give up. They don't know how to take off those added pounds in a hurry so they're discouraged from trying again. This does not normally happen with the Quick Weight Loss Diet because the dieter soon is aware of the fact that his fat *can* come off in a hurry—*it has happened to him.*

2. HOW THE QUICK WEIGHT
LOSS METHOD WORKS

The Quick Weight Loss Diet has built into it elements to reduce you even by subterfuge. For example, there is no instruction to count calories. You can eat as much of the fine foods on the list as you need to satisfy your hunger: a great variety of lean meats, unfatty fish and seafood, chicken and turkey, eggs, cottage cheese and farmer cheese.

Your first reaction may well be that of so many of my patients, "But on that diet I'll eat my head off. I'll consume far more calories than I do now." The fact is that on this diet, even eating 6 or more meals a day, you'll find that you limit the intake yourself because you feel full and lack the desire for excess quantities that would increase your weight instead of taking it off. Also you're restricted from the rich foods that tempt you to overeat. And you eat to satisfy your hunger, not to pamper your appetite. A very few overeat for the first day or two but then taper off quickly.

Many of my patients have told me, "I feel I'm eating so much on that diet, how am I losing so much weight?" When I added up their daily intake I found that they had consumed as few as 400 to 900 calories a day, without any desire for more food. Others, primarily taller persons, were eating up to 2,000 calories a day on the Quick Weight Loss Diet and yet lost pounds rapidly although they hadn't been able to lose on other diets where they seemed to be eating less. The high protein consumption burned up many more calories per day.

With this method, the time comes eventually when you are either at or near your ideal weight. For the average person who is reducing drastically, it is best to come within 5 to 15 pounds of the ideal weight, then go on Stay Slim Eating for a few months. After that you take off the remaining 5 to 15 excess pounds through the Quick Weight Loss Diet, then back to Stay Slim Eating when your ideal weight is achieved.

Here are just a very few typical records of how individuals reduced with the aid of this method. In every one of these successful cases and thousands more, not one patient showed any harmful effects. Every one improved his or her health and well-being by losing excess weight. The usual comment: "Doctor, I feel wonderful. I have new energy. Everything looks brighter. My husband and friends tell me that I look years younger and far more attractive."

One of my patients is a physician who was considerably overweight. She is 5′ 3½″ and weighed 183 pounds. I placed her on the Quick Weight Loss Diet, prescribed medication and told her to eat only if hungry. She never stopped her practice as a busy doctor. On her own decision, she went for 7 days on water and vitamins, starting on my diet only from the eighth day. She lost 13 pounds the first week, 12 pounds the second week, 6 pounds the third week—dropping from 183 to 152 pounds, 31 pounds in 3 weeks. She will continue to diet until she stabilizes at 125 pounds, then will go down eventually to 110 pounds, about her ideal weight. Her opinion of the Quick Weight Loss Diet: "It's great!"

QUICK WEIGHT LOSS FOR FAMILIES

Entire families lose pounds wonderfully through the Quick Weight Loss Diet (it usually helps when two or more people go on the diet together and, in effect, have a contest with each other). In one instance of a family of four, during the first four days on the diet the considerably overweight father dropped nine pounds. Mother, only a few pounds overweight after a heavy-eating cruise, lost the four pounds she'd gained on vacation. The 14-year-old overweight daughter dropped six pounds. Even the average-weight 16-year-old son who was not on the diet itself went down a pound, influenced by the way the others were eating.

They were all so delighted that the two overweights continued dieting and losing weight. The happiest result was that the father, who had never been able to stick with a diet before, reduced to a slim, attractive figure his children had never seen. He'd given up that goal many years before as unattainable for the rest of his life. One doctor after another had told him to reduce for his health's sake but he hadn't succeeded.

The family called the diet a "miracle." Actually it was just another proof of the sound functioning of the quick reducing method. People need specific instructions that work, not outmoded reducing theories amounting to a recommendation to "eat less"—which are bound to fail for most.

SOME TYPICAL CASES ON THE QUICK WEIGHT LOSS DIET

A.B.—man, 5′ 4″. He weighed 170 pounds and despaired of being able to reduce as he had failed many times. I recommended that he come down to 125–130 pounds, ideal weight for him. On my diet, he lost 7 pounds the first week. His rate of loss varied because of lapses in dieting, but he was down to 127 pounds in 3 months, a loss of 43 pounds and at ideal weight. He felt so good that he had refused to stop dieting on the way down, and he continued to cut down for another 6 weeks until he weighed 116 pounds.

I emphasized that there was no advantage to him in being underweight so during the next month he rose to 127 pounds. Gradually, not taking care in following the Combination Plan, over the next 4 months he

A.B.—man 5′ 4″ tall—one year record

went up to 138 pounds. Going back on the Quick
Weight Loss Diet which he had learned was relatively
easy, he then reduced within a month to 128 pounds
where his weight has now been stabilized for some
time, as charted.

B.C.—woman, 5′ 3″. She weighed 147 pounds, over
30 pounds heavier than her ideal weight of 103–115.
On the Quick Weight Loss Diet, she dropped 6 pounds
the first week and was down to 130 pounds in 6 weeks.
I told her to maintain that weight for a few weeks,
then go down to 120 and stay there for six months before stabilizing at about 110. We both knew she could
do it because she had learned how relatively easy it
had been to take off over 25 pounds.

C.C.—woman, 5′ 5″. She weighed 174 pounds, dragging around a load of about 50 pounds more than her
ideal weight of under 125. She told me, "Doctor, I feel
terrible in every way. I've tried to diet gradually but

it doesn't work for me." I started her on the Quick Weight Loss Diet and also prescribed a drug for assistance. At the end of a week she had lost 10 pounds and was down to 164.

"I'm feeling so much better already," she told me, "that nothing can stop me now from getting down to normal weight. When I lost a few pounds the first week on other diets, it didn't mean anything to me, but 10 pounds—that really proves something. My husband said I'll soon be looking like his bride again." Eventually she reached her ideal weight.

D.E.—man, 5′ 11″. He weighed 243 pounds instead of between 153 and 170 pounds ideal weight. He had high blood pressure and many other undesirable symptoms and ills. He said he felt like an old man although he was only 32. On my diet he went down to 183 pounds over a period of 14 weeks. His blood pressure dropped from 210/135 to 150/100. He will be on Stay Slim Eating for a while and then will lose 20 to 25 pounds, stabilizing at about 165. With the big weight loss already, he says that he feels like "a new man."

E.F.—woman, 5′ 2″. She weighed 155 pounds instead of her ideal weight of under 110. She said she was determined to take off weight because she heard someone refer to her as a "butterball." In 2 months on the Quick Weight Loss Diet she was down to 115 pounds. Letting up too much, her weight rose to 124 pounds in a month. On the Quick Loss Diet she dropped to 115 pounds in 2 weeks and then to 110.

She asked me, "Will I have to be careful about how much I eat for the rest of my life?" "Yes," I told her, "just like millions of others who are anxious to stay thin, healthy, vigorous and attractive. Isn't it worth the difference in the way you look and feel now?" She agreed that it was. She is proving it by maintaining her ideal weight on the Combination Plan, return-

ing to the Quick Loss Diet for brief periods whenever
her weight rises, which is seldom.

F.G.—woman, 5′ 1″. She weighed 194 pounds and
said that she had tried to reduce *fourteen* different
times without success. Each time she had lost a few
pounds and then gained the weight right back again.
By the Quick Loss method, she lost over 10 pounds the
first week. She was so encouraged that she continued
eagerly. Within a year she was at her desired weight
of under 105 pounds and has maintained this for over
4 years at this writing.

In typical cases like the preceding, the loss of weight
takes dangerous strain off the heart. I'm often asked,
"Doesn't such dieting put a great strain on the heart
due to the sudden change?" The answer is precisely
the opposite; taking off excess fat takes strain off the
heart. The electrocardiograms (on page 21) of an average individual show how this becomes apparent.

With the aid of quick loss dieting, years of life were
undoubtedly added for this patient. Dangerous heart
impairment from overweight was avoided. The fat
crowding the organs was eliminated. The organs returned to normal and the signs of heart strain disappeared.

(1) The first simplified graph depicts an electrocardiogram at normal weight with what is known as the T-wave rounded or peaked as here:

(2) As the person gains weight, the T-wave is slightly flattened:

(3) With further gain of weight, the T-wave has disappeared, a clear warning that heart strain is imminent:

(4) The person has now put on additional weight, is considerably overweight and the T-wave is inverted, a certain sign of heart strain that can be serious:

(5) Fortunately the individual was warned to diet or possibly incur serious heart damage. As the weight came off, the T-wave direction was reversed and the inverted line flattened:

(6) With further loss, the T-wave peak began to appear again:

(7) With successful dieting, at desired weight, the T-wave is peaked again, the danger signal of heart strain gone:

3. THE GOAL: YOUR IDEAL WEIGHT

The Quick Weight Loss Diet will help you attain your ideal weight quickly. This "ideal weight table" based on my findings differs from others. I don't believe that you should be guided by what the average weight is for persons of your height but rather by what your ideal weight should be for maximum health, well-being and long life. The average weights listed by others are often too high, in my opinion, because too many Americans are overweight and this raises the averages above the ideal weight.

I don't give figures by "type of frame" because this is misleading to many. What comprises a small, medium or large frame isn't easy for the individual to decide for himself. Nearly all my overweight patients have claimed to have large bone structure although only a small percentage were in that category. Very few chose to consider themselves as having a small frame because it would mean that their weight should be even lower.

There are too many variations for you to be able to determine correctly what kind of frame and bone structure category fits you. Many people have broad shoulders and a small pelvis. Others have just the opposite. Some have a thin chest and heavy legs and thighs. Some have short, thick necks but with thin hands and arms, and large feet and legs—or just the opposite.

I recommend that you aim for your weight listed on the following Weight and Daily Calorie Table, a few pounds one way or the other; lower is better than higher. The lower figure is the "ideal weight" (which may be called "desirable weight" by some statisticians or doctors). The higher figure is the "average weight" for the height. These figures are for men and women aged 25 and over, in stockinged feet, and without jackets. Note also your daily calorie intake to maintain ideal weight.

WEIGHT AND DAILY CALORIE TABLE

	Women			Men	
Weight	Daily Calorie Intake	Height	Weight	Daily Calorie Intake	
95–100	1,200–1,500	5′	105–110	1,320–1,650	
95–105	1,260–1,575	5′ 1″	105–115	1,390–1,735	
100–110	1,320–1,650	5′ 2″	110–121	1,450–1,815	
103–115	1,380–1,725	5′ 3″	113–126	1,520–1,900	
108–120	1,440–1,800	5′ 4″	120–132	1,585–1,980	
112–125	1,500–1,875	5′ 5″	123–137	1,650–2,065	
117–130	1,560–1,950	5′ 6″	130–143	1,715–2,145	
121–135	1,620–2,025	5′ 7″	133–148	1,780–2,230	
124–140	1,680–2,100	5′ 8″	140–154	1,850–2,310	
130–145	1,740–2,175	5′ 9″	143–159	1,915–2,400	
135–150	1,800–2,250	5′ 10″	150–165	1,980–2,475	
140–155	1,860–2,325	5′ 11″	153–170	2,045–2,560	
144–160	1,920–2,400	6′	160–176	2,110–2,640	
148–165	1,980–2,475	6′ 1″	163–181	2,180–2,725	
153–170	2,040–2,500	6′ 2″	170–187	2,245–2,800	

The preceding weight table is figured generally as follows:

WOMEN aged 25 or over: 5 feet—100 pounds. For every inch above 5 feet, add 5 pounds per inch for average weight; from that figure subtract about 10 percent for ideal weight; the figures give you the range between ideal and average weight as a guide. For 18 to 25 years of age, subtract 1 pound for each year under 25. For example, a girl of 19, 5′ 4″ tall, ideal weight—102 pounds, average weight—114 pounds.

MEN aged 25 or over: 5 feet—110 pounds. For

every inch over 5 feet, add 5½ pounds per inch for average weight; from that figure subtract about 10% for ideal weight; the figures give you the range between ideal and average weight as a guide. For 18 to 25 years of age, subtract 1 pound for each year under 25. For example, a young man of 21, 5′ 10″ tall, ideal weight—146 pounds, average weight—161 pounds.

ADDED SUGGESTIONS: If you're a professional in the theatrical or entertainment fields, a clothes model, an athlete or a dancer, it is best that your weight be about 5 pounds less than the ideal weights listed.

If you have been considerably overweight for years, I recommend that you reduce with the Quick Weight Loss Diet to within 5 to 15 pounds of the average weight for your height. After maintaining that figure for six months to a year, I suggest that you reduce further to your ideal weight and maintain it thereafter.

CALORIE INTAKE: If you wish to calculate your daily calorie intake according to the average weight for your height, figure 12 to 15 calories per pound.

For example, if the average weight for your height according to the preceding table is 120 pounds: 120 $\times$ 12 $=$ 1,440 calories; 120 $\times$ 15 $=$ 1,800 calories. Your calorie intake to maintain that weight would be 1,440 to 1,800 daily. In reducing, you add up everything and eat 1,440 to 1,800 calories daily (if you're overweight you're now consuming many more calories than that). But this type of attempted self-discipline which results usually in slow weight loss rarely works.

INEFFECTIVE BALANCED DIETING IS USELESS

An advertisement for the National Livestock and Meat Board was headlined, "The Secret of Weight Control: Cutting Down—Not Out!" It went on to state, "You don't need to be scientific about what you eat, just sensible . . . and forget about fads. Eat a variety of foods and not too many calories, that's the way to good nutrition. Not a very complicated idea, but a sound one!"

All that is true as far as it goes, which is far short of the reducer's goal. Balanced eating is a very "sensible" system. But for most overweights it just doesn't work. And if it doesn't work for you then the concept of balanced dieting is useless for you because it doesn't take off your excess weight.

There's no question in the minds of these people of *wanting* to be slim. The question is how you can accomplish it realistically and surely. Hundreds, thousands of persons have told me, "Doctor, I've tried to cut down on my eating and on calories but I just can't. I've failed dozens of times." Am I, as a doctor, then supposed to fail my patients?

According to those who advocate balanced eating only, one should say in effect, "I can't help you if you won't regulate your eating and limit yourself to smaller portions of only the foods on a balanced diet list." But I know that most overweights will fail on such advice just as surely as if I said, "No special diet, just balanced eating—and buy your clothes two sizes too big."

I've had to find out over the years, by trial and error, what will help most overweights to reduce, not just what they should do but what they *will* do. Accordingly I've devised these quick loss diets, methods and specific instructions and recommendations. My experience has proved that these techniques work. The pounds come off safely, swiftly and far more surely with the Quick Weight Loss Diet and with the many bizarre quick action diets listed later to accommodate your personal needs.

GET STARTED NOW . . .

I recommend that you start at once with the proved Quick Weight Loss method on which *you don't count calories.* You will lose weight quickly because of the restricted types of foods and other elements which result in your consuming fewer calories and *burning up more calories* than with varied eating.

Please keep this in mind every single day that you're reducing: You are not guessing that the Quick Weight Loss Diet will work. You are not relying on false claims or empty promises. This method has been proved in the cases of many thousands of others who have regained attractive figures. It will work for you—swiftly, pleasantly, surely. Just give the Quick Weight Loss Diet at least one week's trial. Never again will you moan hopelessly in Shakespeare's words: "O! that this too too solid flesh would melt." This time you can have confidence that you'll achieve the wonderful reducing results and the slim figure you want.

4. THE PROVED QUICK
WEIGHT LOSS METHOD

Not only from repeated successes with thousands of men and women, but also from extensive study and analysis of every kind of diet I could find, I'm convinced that the Quick Weight Loss Diet is the finest and best for most people who should take off excess weight. Judging from the records of my patients, if you adhere to this simple, satisfying diet faithfully, *you should expect to lose 5% to 10% of your weight the first week if you are overweight.* If you weigh 150 pounds and are considerably overweight, you should lose between 7 and 15 pounds the first week.

Another way of figuring your probable loss according to the averages is that you should lose 5 pounds a week, week after week. If you are 10 pounds overweight, it should take you 2 weeks to lose that excess. If you're 15 pounds overweight, you'll probably take off that excess weight in only 3 weeks.

There may be weeks when you'll lose 3 pounds or so, and other weeks when you'll drop about 10 pounds. It's not unusual for a considerably overweight person to lose 15 to 25 pounds the first week (25 pounds being about the greatest loss in a week on my records with the Quick Weight Loss Diet, as previously noted).

You score these satisfying losses while you eat excellent wholesome foods on this diet—lean meats, fish, poultry, sea food, eggs, cottage cheese, farmer cheese. You can have as much coffee and tea as desired, without sugar or cream or milk but with non-caloric sweeteners if you like. You may drink as many non-caloric carbonated beverages as you wish.

You'll note definite "must" restrictions on the diet but most of my patients have not found them too limiting or difficult. Right from the start you take off excess fat quickly to reach your desired weight. Then you may indulge yourself in the foods you enjoy most, within reason. It's important that you weigh yourself every morning. If you see that you're 3 pounds or more above your ideal weight, back you go on the Quick Loss Diet for a week to burn off unwanted fat. Each time you go back on the diet you'll find it easier to maintain your ideal weight afterwards.

THE QUICK LOSS METHOD

Eat all you wish of the following foods to satisfy hunger. If you eat until you've satisfied your hunger but haven't stuffed yourself, and then feel hungry before the next meal, you can eat again but only from the foods listed here. In fact, you're better off eating smaller meals 6 times a day than 3 bigger meals as is the general custom. But you limit yourself to this extensive selection of high protein foods.

1. LEAN MEATS, with all possible fat trimmed off. Includes beef, lamb, veal. Eat it broiled, boiled, baked or smoked. No butter, margarine, oil or other fats or greases are to be used either in the cooking or in the eating.

2. CHICKEN AND TURKEY with all skin removed. Broiled, boiled or roasted, with no butter, margarine, oil or other fats or greases. Young fowl is preferable but not necessary.

3. ALL LEAN FISH such as flounder, haddock, cod, perch; SEA FOOD: shrimps, scallops, lobsters, oysters, clams, crabs. Broiled, baked or boiled. No butter, margarine, oil or other fats or greases permitted in preparation or in serving. You may have cocktail sauce, horseradish, ketchup—in moderation.

4. EGGS. Hard boiled preferably. Also soft or medium boiled eggs, poached or any type of fried eggs made in non-fat, non-stick pans without butter, margarine, oil or other fats or greases.

5. COTTAGE CHEESE, FARMER CHEESE, POT CHEESE and other cheeses made with skim milk and no whole milk.

6. AT LEAST 8 GLASSES OF WATER DAILY, absolutely essential (10-ounce glasses). As much as you want of coffee and tea without cream, milk or sugar. You may sweeten with non-caloric sugar substitutes to taste. Enjoy all the club soda, vichy and non-caloric carbonated beverages you wish, as often as desired.

The eight glasses of water daily are in addition to whatever coffee, tea and non-caloric carbonated beverages you drink. This is an integral part of the specific internal process put into motion by the Quick Weight Loss Diet. Much more of your body fat is burned up than with most other diets. This leaves in its wake the waste products or ashes of burnt fat. They must all be washed out of your system by water which also serves to relieve any unpleasant dryness and taste in the mouth.

Any time you feel a great desire for sweets, pour a glassful of non-caloric carbonated beverage, varying the flavors you like most. This is a treat you may enjoy just about as many times a day as you wish. Such drinks are refreshing and satisfying to your "sweet tooth." They contain no carbohydrates and add to the desired flow of liquids through your system.

You may use common seasonings such as salt, pepper, garlic, cloves, thyme, other herbs and spices, cocktail sauce, tabasco sauce, horseradish, ketchup. Don't use any creamy or oily sauces or dressings. No mayonnaise, no salad dressings, no oils, no fats.

It is desirable to take vitamins daily with the diet, such as a once-daily vitamin and mineral tablet which contains vitamins A (5,000 USP units), D (500 units), B-1 (3 mg.), B-2 (3 mg.), C (50 mg.), and additional varied vitamins and minerals. (I don't recommend any particular brand or this formula specifically —most any once-daily vitamin will do, with varying contents of vitamins and minerals, as offered by many different companies.) If you're very much determined to lose weight rapidly, and you cut down your eating to a minimum on the Quick Loss Diet, take 2 of the once-daily vitamin tablets each day, or choose commonly available "therapeutic" tablets or capsules containing higher dosages.

NOTHING ELSE IS PERMITTED ON THIS DIET —NOTHING! IF IT'S NOT MENTIONED IN THE PRECEDING LIST, DON'T EAT IT OR DRINK IT. The addition of any other food or drink will prevent the full and efficient functioning of the high protein internal reducing process which burns up more fat.

You'll find that this is a relatively easy diet to maintain when you eat out at restaurants. For example, at a restaurant you can always get broiled, roasted or boiled meat, chicken or fish, sea food, boiled or poached eggs, cottage cheese. You might start with a shrimp cocktail, complete with cocktail sauce. Simply skip the side dishes and eat as much steak or lean hamburger as you wish, for instance, to satisfy your hunger—then stop.

If you're dining at someone's home, carry your Quick Weight Loss Diet listing and show it to your hostess. She should certainly honor your need and resolve to take off dangerous excess weight and not be offended that you don't eat her rich desserts or other foods not permitted on the diet.

Like so many others on this diet, you'll probably be pleased to find that soon you don't miss the butter, margarine, oil or other fats commonly used in preparing and eating foods. Rather, the majority of those on this method decide even after they go off the diet that they prefer the clean taste of good food itself, in its more natural flavoring, without calorie-heavy fats added. A typical comment is: "I used to love French fries but now I can't even stand the thought of them. Give me a clean, naturally tasty, unbuttered baked potato instead any time."

ONLY HALF A GLASS OF WATER PER HOUR

Oddly enough, one of the common reactions I get from people when I recommend the Quick Loss Diet is, "The variety of fine foods sounds wonderful, and all I can eat too, but how can I manage to drink eight glasses of water every day?"

I asked one woman, "Can you drink half a glass of water each waking hour?"

"Of course! Who can't drink half a glass of water an hour?"

"Or, a glass of water every 2 hours?"

"Certainly. Nothing difficult about that."

"Then," I concluded, "what's your concern about being able to drink eight glasses of water a day?"

"Oh . . . I didn't understand. The first thing that entered my head was that I'd have to drink eight glasses of water all at one time . . ."

Was that your first reaction too? If so, it's because your approach to any kind of dieting is negative rather than positive. The first step in taking off that fat and flab is to want to very much, so that you'll start this diet at once and stay with it at least a full week. I know three overweight roommates, young women, who started this diet together and lost 14, 15 and 17 pounds respectively the first week.

Figure out right now how much less you'll weigh at the end of one week. Isn't that a worthwhile goal? Practically any obstacles can be overcome if you care enough. Patients who are not near a convenient supply of water at all times, such as taxicab drivers, carry a jug of cold water with them.

Try the Quick Loss method for a week positively, optimistically, not negatively as though you're depriving yourself of anything important. As I told an over-weight patient (F.G.), "You worry about drinking eight glasses of water a day as a great chore. Yet you have no trouble at all stuffing your fat-choked insides each day with dish after dish of rich heavy food, ruining your health and shortening your life."

She ran to the water tap in a hurry, started on the Quick Loss Diet right there and then. She dropped from 161 to 151, a loss of 10 pounds, the first week. In 6 weeks she weighed 135 pounds, 26 pounds taken off in that brief period. She is headed for her ideal weight of 120 pounds.

PROVED SUPERIOR BY THOUSANDS . . .

One of the best features of this method, as I have learned from its use by thousands of individuals, is the enthusiasm it arouses among those following it. Practically all have found it "easy to take." The drop shown on the scale each morning spurs them to stay within the simple specifications instead of giving up as they had on so many diets so many times before.

With this diet you eat all you want from the foods on the list, enough to satisfy your hunger but not in excess just for eating pleasure. This is in effect a "demand diet" in that you eat whenever your hunger demands. It is also a form of "nibbler's diet" since you eat just enough to satisfy yourself and only when you're hungry.

You'll find that you're not as tempted to overeat the foods on the Quick Loss Diet as you are by rich, starchy, sweet, calorie-heavy dishes you might stuff yourself with otherwise. You should not overeat at any time. Stop when you've satisfied your hunger and you'll lose weight rapidly.

You don't count calories because there's no need to do so, the diet itself is self-limiting in effect. When you have taken off the desired weight and shift to Stay Slim Eating, it is then advisable to learn the calorie value of foods and restrict yourself to 1700 to 2500 calories daily (for men) or 1300 to 2200 calories per day (for women).

To sum up, the Quick Loss Diet has helped more people in my care take off up to 50 pounds of excess weight and keep it off than any other dieting program I know of.

The diet is listed below in brief format. I suggest that you make two copies of it. Pin up one copy of the listing in your kitchen so you'll have it there for constant reminder and reference. Carry the other copy in your pocket or purse for reference if you eat out.

THE QUICK WEIGHT LOSS DIET—eat only food on this listing:

1. LEAN MEATS—boiled, baked or broiled—no butter, margarine, oil or other fats

2. CHICKEN, TURKEY—all skin removed— broiled, boiled or roasted—no butter, margarine, oil, fats

3. LEAN FISH, SEA FOOD—broiled, boiled or baked. No butter, margarine, oil, fats. Cocktail sauce, ketchup, horseradish, all permitted in moderation

4. EGGS—preferably hard-boiled, but also may be cooked any way not using butter, margarine, oil, fats

5. COTTAGE CHEESE, FARMER CHEESE, POT CHEESE, SKIM MILK CHEESES.

6. AT LEAST 8 GLASSES OF WATER DAILY ESSENTIAL! As much as you want of coffee, tea (without cream, milk, sugar), club soda, vichy, non-caloric carbonated beverages. Non-caloric sugar substitutes permitted

You may use common seasonings such as salt, pepper, spices, cocktail sauce, ketchup, horseradish.

NOTHING ELSE PERMITTED—IF IT'S NOT LISTED HERE, DON'T EAT OR DRINK IT!

5. HOW THIS DIET BURNS UP 275 MORE CALORIES DAILY

If you're concerned only with the "how" of taking off excess weight rapidly, then you can simply use the Quick Weight Loss Diet and get its benefits. You need not read the details here on "why" this high protein diet functions so well in the human system to reduce you faster. This information is for those who are interested and who find it helps them to keep dieting when they know such "whys."

This explanation is in the most simplified terms, certainly not in complete scientific detail which only scholars would understand—they know all this already. The diet is made up entirely of protein, chief constituent of animal bodies. The ability of protein to produce more energy is called the specific dynamic action of protein.

What is important to you is that this diet, which in essence provides protein only, works more efficiently than other types of diets, from a chemical and metabolic viewpoint, in burning up fat. With this method, the system burns up about 275 more calories daily than a diet of the same total caloric intake but including, for example, fruits, vegetables, butter, margarine and oil.

Most foods that grow have some protein in them and are able to raise the fires of metabolism to some extent. The degree depends on the amount of protein in the foods. Those listed on the Quick Loss Diet have a higher proportion of protein. The resultant burning capacity is excellent so that you eat and burn up your own fat. Some of this fat (your own body fat) is converted into a small amount of carbohydrate or sugar. The remainder of the fat is converted into energy or fuel. The fat is mainly broken down into fatty acids which provide the body with its heat and energy when no carbohydrates or sugars are ingested. This process is a step by step reaction; with each reaction some energy and heat are slowly given off.

In this process, about 60% of the fat is completely oxidized (united with oxygen) into carbon dioxide and water. A large percentage is left as ashes in the "furnace" to be disposed of. (Unused fatty acids such as oxybutyric acid and aceto-acetic acid are the "ashes" of fat refuse.)

Studies have shown that persons on a high protein diet such as this, with no carbohydrate intake, melt the fat out of the storage or fat centers. The fat is brought to the blood where it is transported to the liver. Here it is broken down into bile salts and acids. The unused fat is again poured into the blood as ketone bodies.

These are really fatty acids which are brought to the kidneys and carried away in the urine. The body withdraws extra water to dilute these acids. That is why the body not only loses extra fat but also depletes extra intercellular water and is a reason why there is usually more frequent urination with this diet. As a result, the body is lighter, and the heart, lungs and blood vessels beat, breathe and flow more easily. Thus most people on the diet feel lighter and better very quickly.

The fatty acids are also slight irritants to the kidney. In order to get rid of them the body must have plenty of water to wash them out. That's why no less than 8 glasses of water a day are specified.

If you should take sugars and carbohydrates, here is why it would cut down radically the effectiveness of the Quick Loss Diet. Each gram of carbohydrate you ingest substitutes for the burning up of 1 to 2 grams of your body fat, equivalent to 9 or 18 calories. If carbohydrates are taken in, the body ignores using its fat and uses the carbohydrates only. Thus the fat, instead of being burned up, is stored in your fat depots.

The "why" of this functioning is not fully understood scientifically. But on this regiment, you as a dieter get the advantage of this fact and continue to reduce even though you may be eating permitted protein foods totaling 1,300 to 2,500 calories daily.

If you disregard the instructions and eat regular carbohydrates or sugar or alcohol, you will stop burning up stored fat as efficiently. Even one indiscretion, one mouthful of ice cream, for example, will set you back a day or two. The diet must be observed strictly or you will not do as well as many thousands before you have done in using up bulging fat.

You will lose the most weight on the Quick Loss Diet, most quickly, if you eat only to satisfy your hunger pangs rather than to gratify a desire to eat just for the pleasure of eating. Understand that with this diet your body supplies the fat and carbohydrates which are lacking in the diet. You use up stored fat for energy and also convert the protein into starches for energy. So the less you eat, the more you use up excess fat stored in your body.

I must make it clear from a professional viewpoint that the Quick Loss Diet is not a "miracle cure" or a scientific functioning of my invention. High-protein diets are not "new"; this is my own version, one which I have found to be most usable and effective.

THIS QUICK WEIGHT LOSS IS NOT MOSTLY WATER LOSS

Again and again I hear ignorant people, mostly heavyweights who resist dieting, say, "Quick dieting weight loss is phony—it's mostly water loss. You dump a lot of water the first few days and then the weight comes back." That is nonsense in respect to my method.

I've had patient after patient lose a great deal of weight the first week and then 5 to 6 pounds consistently week after week on this diet. While some of this weight loss is water, even the worst diehard must admit that most of it is excess body fat.

Consider the case of a patient, a very heavy man, who lost 112 pounds in 16 weeks on a particularly limited version of this method. He felt fine all the way as he dropped from 354 to 242 pounds. He ate only 1 meal a day when he felt hungry, at no set hour. He drank a great deal of water and club soda as he put in a long, hard week's work week after week.

He had no ailments or complaints and never felt weak or exhausted. He slept well. His blood pressure which had been much too high dropped to normal. Since he reached his desired weight he has had no difficulty maintaining it.

Here's the week-by-week record of this man's weight loss:

1st week—17 lbs.	5th— 4	9th— 2	13th—8
2nd " —10	6th— 6	10th—11	14th—5
3rd " — 6	7th— 6	11th— 4	15th—6
4th " — 7	8th—13	12th— 1	16th—6

This loss of 112 pounds certainly was not all water. Nor are the losses by hundreds upon hundreds of individuals whom I've watched drop 40 to 75 pounds and maintain the reduced weight. These people were not waterlogged nor are you unless you have some disorder which your doctor has already noted.

So I suggest that you stop worrying about losing only water. Instead, start Quick Weight Loss dieting. As your clothes become sizes too big for you, you'll agree that you've melted off pounds and inches of all too solid, unhealthy and unwanted flesh, not water.

WHAT NOT TO EAT

Your simple guide is to eat only the foods previously listed. Remember, you follow these restrictions for a limited time, not forever. As examples, here are some foods not allowed: No bread, rolls or cake in any form. No vegetables, not even lettuce or celery. No fruits of any kind, no oranges, lemons or grapefruit in solid form or in juices.

No medical "fillers" such as methyl cellulose which I'm sure doesn't sound very appetizing to you anyhow.

No alcohol is permitted for the duration of the diet; no Scotch, whiskey, gin, or even the driest wines or beer. You can have these drinks in moderation, and your favorite foods in moderate portions, after you reach your ideal weight.

No ice cream, ices, sherbets or the like, no desserts.

No soft drinks containing sugar. You can drink and enjoy all the non-caloric carbonated beverages you wish, as much as you want. If you take a blindfold test, you won't be able to taste the difference between sodas made with sugar and those made with non-caloric sugar substitutes.

No dairy products outside of the eggs and a few cheeses mentioned in the listing. No whole milk or cream. No sugar in coffee or tea; use as much as you want of the non-caloric sweeteners, in liquid, tablet, powder or other form.

Don't allow yourself even such seemingly small indulgences as taking a few candy mints, fruit drops, other small sweets or chewing gum while you're on this diet. The reason is that you may well be one of the many persons who cannot metabolize carbohydrates properly. Even the relatively small quantity of carbohydrates in a candy mint or stick of gum seems to be converted into fat in the system rather than burned up for energy and heat. That slight amount disturbs the adjustment in the body whereby the functioning of the Quick Loss Diet burns up fat most efficiently.

The same applies to bread, cake, cookies, jelly, cereals, noodles, alcoholic beverages, or any of the hundreds of products which contain the slightest amounts of carbohydrates. Don't eat even a tiny cookie or sip a small alcoholic drink or you'll throw the entire reducing process out of kilter.

In short, if a food is not on the listing, and you question whether or not you're allowed to eat it, the answer is "No!"

Most of my patients haven't found the restrictions too hard to handle because they realize that they can indulge in such foods and drinks in moderation once they lose their excess weight. They know, as you will, that you go on this diet "for a limited time only."

WELL-BEING ON THE QUICK LOSS DIET

The vast majority of people on this diet feel normal and perfectly well physically. Many have told me they felt particularly happy, alert, vigorous and in high spirits.

For the great majority of persons, the Quick Loss Diet provides all the protein needed, all the fat and vitamins required by the system. There would seem to be a lack of vitamin C on this diet but it's actually provided by the fresh fish, sea food and meat. In all my observations, I've never found one person who has developed a clinical vitamin deficiency on this diet. Nevertheless I recommend that you take a once-daily vitamin which supplies the supposedly normal daily vitamin requirement.

Remember that patients of mine have lost as much as 25 pounds the first week and 106 pounds in 3 months on this diet. Thorough examination of these persons and many others did not disclose any undesirable neurological or physical signs, no vitamin deficiency. It is good medical practice to have your doc-

tor examine you occasionally while on this diet or any
diet.

REGARDING WASTE ELIMINATION

This diet has practically no residue. Therefore it
is likely that you may not have a bowel movement for
a few days, although not necessarily so. In any case,
don't be disturbed by any such lack. If you are at
all concerned, take some mineral oil or milk of magnesia. Nature adjusts the bowel habits so that many
persons soon have a daily movement again in spite
of the lessened residue.

Protein produces a different intestinal flora or
bacterial growth. As a result, many patients have told
me that they have a new surge of well-being within a
surprisingly short time. Many of them quickly lost the
bloated abdominal feeling which they'd borne while
overweight.

The Quick Loss Diet is also excellent in that the
individual usually loses a great deal of water. You'll
find that urination increases, often considerably as
water and fats and waste are removed from your
body. I've had some patients on this diet lose over
10 pounds of water in a week. *You are also losing
considerable fat at the same time*.

Women who retain water on this diet and do not
give it up readily usually are about to have a period,
or seem to retain water for some unknown reason. If
they are among the rare few who have low protein
in the blood, they are already aware of it. They
should diet under the direction of a doctor. He will
prescribe one of many diuretics which will be of assistance in such cases. Eliminating salt from the diet
also helps those who retain water.

ADDITIONAL POINTS

Since you are an individual and no two persons are exactly alike, you may apply variations of the diet as noted here.

If you're allergic to eggs, don't eat any—it's unnecessary. The listing shows what you're permitted to eat, not what you must eat.

If your cholesterol count is high (as your doctor would have informed you in the past), don't eat more than four eggs a week.

If you're allergic to shellfish, omit only those species which affect you adversely. Eat the others, also lean fish.

You may eat creamed cottage cheese which is usually the easiest to get. If your cholesterol is high, use pot cheese and farmer cheese to which no milk has been added to make it "creamed."

After you've been on the Quick Weight Loss Diet for some time and taken off more than 30 pounds, you may add moderate portions of artificially sweetened gelatin, plain yogurt, skim milk. However, you will lose faster if you don't add these foods.

As with all reducing diets, I suggest that you have no more than eight hours of sleep daily with this method. When you sleep more than eight hours, you're not assisting your body to burn up food most effectively and helpfully. You'll make reducing easier by keeping active and alert, on the go rather than on your back sleeping.

There's always a question in medical practice whether or not to tell a patient who is on a restricted diet what unusual sensations or symptoms may crop up in a very small percentage of cases. With a very impressionable person the doctor always runs the risk that such complaints may be introduced unknowingly even if they don't exist.

Another risk the doctor faces is that signs and

symptoms may appear which are not imaginary but
real and may be concealed by the patient because
he is so anxious to reduce and doesn't want anything to slow him up. Therefore even though a high
percentage of complaints are unfounded or imagined,
I must list those that do occur although very few individuals are so affected.

I've already mentioned dry, unpleasant taste in the
mouth and on the breath which may occur if you don't
drink at least 8 glasses of water a day. Just drink
enough water and this will not happen, also the diet
will work most efficiently.

A very few people on the diet report some slight
fatigue, a tired and sleepy feeling. This is readily
corrected by a little quiet rest. Some very active
people have said that they seem to lose some of their
pep but gain it all back and more after 2 or 3 days.
On the other hand, most people on the diet report
a more buoyant, reenergized feeling almost from the
start of the diet.

Experiments have shown that some individuals on
a diet such as this, free of carbohydrates including
sugars, do not manufacture the necessary sugar from
the protein and fat. While the system in such persons
does change protein to sugar (gluconeogenesis)
and the body does use it, the result is not as effective
as a sugar which comes from actual sugars, fruits,
vegetables and cereals. Accordingly a slight feeling of
fatigue may develop. Such persons will respond immediately by taking a little sugar such as candy or
orange juice, and any fatigue will vanish. If the
fatigue keeps recurring, switch to another of the diets
listed later. (The feeling described should not be con-
fused with the weak, trembly, perspiring symptoms
due to a low blood sugar which a doctor's examination should reveal and which he would then treat accordingly.)

A very few persons on the diet say that the first
day or two they've felt a slight lightheadedness or

giddy sensation on arising from lying down. This may be due to a drop in blood pressure or loss of sugar, water, or salt. This is rectified by arising slowly rather than rapidly from a horizontal or sitting position. I've found that such symptoms, if real, are very fleeting and invariably disappear after the first day or two on the diet.

It is vital to emphasize again that undesirable symptoms are *rare* among the many patients I've checked on this diet.

6. COMBINATION PLAN KEEPS WEIGHT DOWN: QUICK WEIGHT LOSS AND STAY SLIM EATING

With the Quick Weight Loss method, followed as instructed, you will attain your desired or ideal weight. Now the problem arises, how can I keep my weight down? How can I prevent that dangerous excess fat from creeping up on me again?

The combination of varied Stay Slim Eating and occasional return to Quick Loss dieting, if necessary, has made staying slim a happier, healthier way of living for thousands of women and men. It can do the same for you pleasantly and practicably.

Make no mistake about this—you do not go back to the eating habits that made you fat before. You must keep watching your weight. The happy surprise is that the techniques which have resulted in your losing weight make it easier to maintain ideal weight.

Instead of going on an eating binge after the diet, as some of my patients might have expected, they discovered that they had lost much of their exaggerated desire for rich foods and overeating. You don't have as much trouble fighting temptation because that driving hunger has diminished.

Furthermore the majority of my dieters, and most hopefully you too, realize that as dependence on food and meals diminishes, your other pleasures increase. You usually become more aware that there is greater joy in other activities, in work and in play, in awareness of the world around you, in the physical pleasures of walking, looking, seeing. You're often released from such irritations and chronic ills as indigestion, lethargy, restricted movement, shortness of breath and other common symptoms of overweight. (Note well however that while weight loss is a great aid, it is not a cure-all. Any continuing aches, pains or irregularities should mean a visit to a doctor without delay lest you by-pass urgently needed treatment for some ailment not due specifically to overweight.) Not the least reward you get from this reducing is the surge of pride in your proved willpower. These all-important assets, plus your now habitually decreased appetite, help you form the habit of effective Stay Slim Eating that keeps your weight down. You also keep benefiting from the Quick Loss method for the rest of your life by using it intermittently when necessary.

WATCH THE 3-POUND DANGER SIGNAL

This is primary advice to put into effect to maintain desired slimness. Get on an accurate bathroom scale unclothed the first thing every morning as surely and regularly as you brush your teeth before breakfast. "The horridest of horror tales . . . is often told by bathroom scales." Any time you see that scale mark 3 pounds more than your desired weight, consider it more serious than if your thermometer showed 3 degrees or more over your nomal temperature.

If you climb past that limiting 3-pound number, don't tell yourself that "I'll go easy next week," or "I'll take it off after a while." Take it off now. Starting that day or the next, go back on the Quick Weight Loss Diet for a week.

Fundamentally your Stay Elim Eating from now on will depend on calorie-counting as specified in this chapter. However, the big difference between this method and usual calorie-counting on "balanced dieting" as urged by others is the combination with the Quick Loss method. This is of utmost importance: *this combination is the crucial asset which turns past failures into future rewarding success.* That vital vari-

ance is why most of my patients have been able to
maintain their ideal weight year after year.

CASE HISTORY

Specific examples of how well this combination dieting works are the cases of my collaborator, Samm
Baker (5′ 10½″, age 56) and his attractive wife, Natalie
(5′ 4″, "Over 40").

A chubby youngster, Samm went off to college at
age 16 and trimmed to his normal weight of 155.
Over the years after college he varied between 155
and 165 by counting calories and limiting his intake
accordingly. By age 54 his weight had crept up to
close to 170 and he varied between 162 and 170 although he wanted to get back to 155 for the sake of
best health and appearance. He attributed his weight-
losing difficulty to the demands of social and business
eating.

Natalie had a serious weight problem as a youngster. Between ages 13 and 17 she weighed 167 pounds,
wore size 42. Her fat was considered "a family characteristic." She hated being fat with all the social
problems involved for a high school girl. Her family
thought that fat was a mark of health and good living. Doctors gave her no support, said lightly that
she'd "grow out of it." Summers at camp she would
lose 10 or 15 pounds, then gain it all back after returning to mother's cooking and urging to "eat, it's
good for you."

When she went off to Radcliffe College she determined to become slim. She invented her own rigorous
diet, living primarily on cola soda and peanut butter crackers, skipping the dormitory meals. On vaca-
tions at home she had to pretend to eat because her
mother was alarmed, then she'd return to her strict
dieting at college. By age 19 she weighed 109 pounds
and wore size 8.

All through this 2-year lopsided dieting she had

never been ill even though she hadn't taken vitamins because the concept for everyday usage had not yet been developed. She had become beautiful, admired and socially popular which is food indeed for a woman at any age.

Through the years of marriage and raising two children she maintained her weight by unceasing calorie-counting as she had "a tendency to be heavy." However, similar to her husband's case, her weight crept up as high as 130 at times (averaging about 125) although she felt best and believed she'd look best at 118. She couldn't get down to 118 on maintenance dieting.

At this point I introduced them to the Quick Weight Loss method for losing weight rapidly. They wrote out the diet, attached the sheet to the wall above their dinette table, and went on it together. Within a week each had lost 7 pounds. They returned to Stay Slim Eating for 3 weeks, then up went the Quick Loss Diet on the wall for another week. After the second week, Samm weighed 155 pounds, Natalie 118 pounds.

They've stayed at about this weight for over 2 years at this writing. Any time they gain over 3 pounds more than desired, they go back on the Quick Loss Diet for from 3 to 7 days. They state that their desires for food have diminished. They both look and feel wonderful (as friends keep telling them), and they find enjoyable Stay Slim Eating "a cinch" combined with the quick reducing diet.

Friends to whom they've introduced this method are just as enthusiastic, even more so when they're heavier to start with. They too find it easier to keep their lower poundage figures with an occasional return to the Quick Loss Diet.

7. HOW TO GET THE STAY SLIM EATING HABIT

From now on, Stay Slim Eating by calorie-counting—consciously or unconsciously—should become part of your way of daily living. It has been said that some people are terrible at counting calories, and have the figures to prove it! I disagree thoroughly with any doctors and nutritionists who state pessimistically that you can't get people to count calories. My patients have disproved this thousands of times when they follow the Combination Plan which so often makes the decisive difference between success or failure.

THESE RECOMMENDATIONS ARE SIMPLE, PRACTICAL, WORKABLE:

1. Determine what your daily calorie intake must be according to the "weight and daily calorie table" in Chapter 3. For example, if you're a woman 5′ 4″ tall, your total is 1,440-1,800 calories daily to maintain desired weight of under 120 pounds.

2. Start at once to get the habit of referring to the calorie tables on following pages to regulate your daily calorie intake.

3. Count the calories of everything you eat during the day, starting from your first food. In the beginning, write the figures on a slip of paper you carry or keep handy, and keep a running total. Stop eating for that day when you've reached the permitted amount. You'll find that soon you plan your day's eating automatically so that you apportion enough of your calories

for when you want them most, at dinner for example.

4. If you must exceed your total one day (because of a special dinner, for instance), deduct the excess from your next day's calorie total. Even if you must go on the fasting diet (Chapter 8) the next day to reach your two-day average, do it—you'll be helping, not harming yourself.

5. If the scale indicates the 3-pound overweight danger signal by the end of any week, go on the Quick Weight Loss Diet for the next week, or for 3, 4 or 5 days.

6. Then, after the Quick Loss interval, you start again with step 1 in this listing. You'll probably find to your intense gratification that the more often and longer you practice this combination, the easier it becomes for you to maintain your ideal weight.

CALORIE KNOWLEDGE BECOMES AN AUTOMATIC SAFETY-VALVE

As with most of my patients who have achieved ideal weight, you're likely to remember the general caloric content of foods after you've been counting calories only a week or two. If your remembrance is off a little now and then, it's not serious.

The tables that follow are your guide rather than a precise mathematical formula. No calorie table can be complete or exactly accurate because there is some variation in the size of portions and individual foods. A "medium orange" (65 calories) is not something turned out to a specific size and weight on a factory production line.

Your judgment must usually determine what is small, medium, large. Your decision should err on the side of conservatism if you're doubtful. If you're not sure whether an orange, or a portion, is medium or large, call it "large" and select the item or reduce the portion to what you can definitely classify as "medium," or use a higher calorie count than for a medium portion.

Keep in mind always that you're kidding yourself to your own detriment if you call a large portion a medium one. You may falsify a calorie total on paper, but your body adds correctly and will turn into fat any extra calories that you omit by fake mathematics.

I realize too that the size of portions as related to calorie count may be less clear than you (and I) would like them in the table. I've simplified and clarified the listings as much as I possibly could. You must contribute your own honest analysis and judgment with portions. "One cup" of canned peaches, for example, refers to 8 ounces, and you must decide how many halves or slices that is. Because of variations in the size of the fruit, it just isn't possible to list "6 canned peach halves" rather than "1 cup."

Similarly, the size of "4 ounces of steak" can be determined by you either by weighing the steak or learning how big a piece makes a pound of steak and taking a portion one-fourth that size. You can judge 1 ounce by package content in many cases, as one-fourth of a 4-ounce package. (If listed in grams, 1 ounce equals 30 grams, 3⅓ ounces equal 100 grams.)

Be sure you count everything you eat and drink as part of your daily total calorie intake. If you have a cocktail, for instance, that's fine—but remember that it must count in your mathematics as much as 150 calories of food. If you eat a lot of hors d'oeuvres at a dinner party, you must add the calories to your day's total.

As in Quick Loss dieting, you can appease your appetite with practically unlimited quantities of black coffee and tea with non-caloric sweetening, with hearty bouillon (see table, 10 calories per cup), sugar-free gelatin dessert (10 calories per half-cup serving) and delicious non-caloric carbonated beverages.

By all means take advantage of the low-calorie foods available now to let you consume more calories in meat, vegetables, fruit and other items that are particularly desirable for you personally. Keep in mind that if you have a 10-calorie sugar-free gelatin dessert instead of a 330-calorie slice of apple pie, that allows you 320 calories or an extra quarter-pound of steak and a baked potato.

Get into the excellent habit of drinking 6 or more glasses of water a day to flush out your system healthfully. If you feel very hungry at meals, make it a custom to have a glass of water, club soda, non-caloric beverage or black coffee or tea *before* the meal. You'll find that you then have less desire to eat more than your daily calorie total permits.

Obviously it's simple to work out your own daily menus with this Stay Slim system of calorie-counting. Also use other dieting techniques detailed later, if desired. For example, suppose you're a woman 5′ 4″ and your daily allowance is 1,700 calories. Here's how you might combine calorie-counting and the Nibbler Diet (Chapter 8) for a day of satisfying eating:

Breakfast: 1 cup orange juice (110), black coffee—110 cals.

10 A.M.: Black coffee or tea, 1 slice toast (60) with 1 tblsp. jam (55)—115 cals.

12 noon: Hamburger (245), 4 asparagus (15), half grapefruit (55), black coffee or tea—315 cals.

4 P.M.: Black coffee, tea or non-caloric soda, 1 slice toast (60) with 1 oz. cottage cheese (30)—90 cals.

7 P.M.: 6 shrimps with cocktail sauce (75), 2 lamb chops (280), baked potato (90), spinach (45), lemon meringue pie (300), black coffee or tea—790 cals.

10 P.M.: 1 glass skim milk (90), 2 graham crackers (55)—145 cals.

With all this food you'd consume 1,565 calories and still be 135 calories under your allowance of 1,700. You wouldn't gain weight, especially by dividing the food into 6 feedings during the day. You could select these foods or any others that you prefer. Make up your own combinations to suit your personal desires, as long as you stay within your Stay Slim limit.

For instance, you could have a martini (150) before dinner and a large wedge of watermelon for dessert (120), eliminating the pie (300).

Keep in mind combining calorie-counting with my other suggested quick-reducing diets for variety, taking advantage of the features of each. For example, if you're tempted by angel cake a la mode, make your entire 300–350 calorie lunch in this case a slice of angel cake (120) topped with a scoop of ice cream (200), along with 2 cups of black coffee. You might have a cup of bouillon (10) first. You still won't gain weight and you needn't worry about any nutritional deficiencies. (This all applies to Stay Slim Eating, not while you're on the Quick Weight Loss Diet.)

CALORIE COUNT LISTING

Although calorie figures can't be entirely accurate, as noted, this listing will serve adequately as a guide for checking and totaling your calorie intake. While all foods can't possibly be included, these calorie counts will help you judge for most foods.

MEATS AND POULTRY

(Most meats and poultry figured here as lean, all visible fat trimmed off, about 60 calories per ounce.)

	cals.
Bacon, fried crisp, 2 slices	95
Beef, roast, lean, 4 oz.	210
Hamburger, lean, broiled, 4 oz.	245
Potpie, 8 oz.	460
Steak, lean, broiled, 4 oz.	235
Bologna, 4" medium slice, each slice	85
Chicken, turkey, broiled, 3 oz.	180
Drumstick and thigh with bone, fried, 5 oz.	275
Frankfurter, 1 medium size	155
Ham, smoked, 3 oz.	290
1 cup	320
Canned, all lean, 2 oz.	170
Lamb, chop, broiled, lean only, 2.5 oz.	140
Leg, lean, 2.5 oz.	130
Pork, roast, lean only, 2.5 oz.	175
Sausage, 4 oz.	340
Tongue, beef, 3 oz.	205
Veal, cutlet, broiled, 3 oz.	185
Roast, lean, 3 oz.	280

FISH AND SHELLFISH

Bluefish, baked, broiled, 3 oz.	135
Clams, medium, each	9
Crabmeat, 3 oz.	90
Haddock, fried, 3 oz.	135
Mackerel, broiled, 3 oz.	200
Oysters, medium, each	12
Salmon, canned, 3 oz. drained	120
Sardines, canned, drained, 3 oz.	180
Shad, baked, 3 oz.	170
Shrimps, medium, each	10
Swordfish, broiled with butter, 3 oz.	150
Tuna, canned, drained, 3 oz.	170

VEGETABLES

Asparagus, medium, each	3.5
Avocado, medium, half	185
Beans, baked and canned types, 1 cup	320
Beets, 1 cup	70
Broccoli, 1 cup	45
Brussels sprouts, 1 cup	60

Cabbage, raw, shredded, 1 cup 25
Cooked, 1 cup 45
Carrots, raw, 5½", each 20
Cooked, 1 cup 45
Cauliflower, cooked, 1 cup 30
Celery, 8" stalk, raw 5
Corn, cooked, 5" ear 65
Canned, 1 cup 170
Cucumbers, 7½" each 25
Lettuce, 5" compact head, 1 lb. 70
2 large leaves 5
Lima beans, 1 cup 150
Mushrooms, 1 cup 30
Onions, raw, 2½" each 50
Cooked, 1 cup 80
Parsley, raw, chopped, 1 tbsp. 1
Peas, fresh, cooked, 1 cup 110
Canned, frozen, drained, 1 cup .. 80
Potatoes, medium, baked, with peel 105
without peel 90
Boiled, medium 90
French-fried, 2" x ½", each 15
Mashed, milk, no butter, 1 cup 145
Chips, 2" medium, each 11
Radishes, raw, medium, each 3

Sauerkraut, drained, 1 cup 30
Spinach and other greens, 1 cup 45
Squash, summer type, 1 cup 35
Winter type, 1 cup 95
String beans, 1 cup .. 35
Sweet potatoes, medium, baked 155
Candied 295
Tomatoes, raw, medium 30
Canned, 1 cup 45
Juice, 1 cup (8 oz.) 50

FRUITS

Apples, raw, medium 70
Juice, 1 cup 125
Applesauce, canned, sweetened, 1 cup 185
Apricots, raw, each .. 20
Canned in syrup, 1 cup 220
Bananas, medium, each 85
Blueberries, blackberries, 1 cup 85
Cantaloupe, 5" medium, half 40
Cherries, 1 cup 65
Cranberry sauce, canned, 1 cup 550
Dates, pitted, 1 cup .. 505
Figs, dried, large 2" x 1", each 60

Fruit Cocktail,
canned, in syrup,
1 cup 195

Grapefruit, 5″ medium, half 55

Juice, fresh, 1 cup 95

Grapes, 1 cup 85

Grape juice, bottled, 1
cup 165

Lemons, medium,
each 20

Oranges, medium,
each 65

Juice, fresh, 1 cup.. 110

Peaches, 2″ medium,
each 35

Canned in syrup,
pitted, 1 cup 200

Pears, 3″ medium,
each 100

Pineapple, fresh,
diced, 1 cup 75

Canned in syrup,
1 cup 205

Plums, 2″ medium,
each 30

Prunes, cooked, unsweetened, each 17

Juice, canned,
1 cup 170

Raisins, dried,
1 cup 460

1 level tablespoon 30

Strawberries, fresh,
1 cup 70

Tangerines, med.
2½″, each 40

Watermelon, 4″ x 8″
wedge 120

DAIRY PRODUCTS, EGGS, FATS, OILS, DRESSINGS

Butter, 1 8-oz. cup
(2 ¼-lb. sticks) 1,605

1 pat or square 50

Cheese, American, 1-
inch cube 70

American, process,
1 oz. 105

Cottage cheese,
creamed, 1 oz. .. 30

Farmer cheese, pot
cheese, 1 oz. 25

Cream cheeze, 1 oz. 105

Roquefort-type,
1 oz. 105

Swiss, 1 oz. 105

Eggs, large, cooked
without fat, each 80

Scrambled, fried
with butter, each 115

White only, raw,
each 20

Yolk only, raw,
each 60

Milk (cow's), whole,
1 cup (8 oz.) 165

Skim, nonfat, 1 cup 90

Buttermilk, cultured, 1 cup 90

Cream, light, 1 cup 525

″ 1 tablespoon 35

″ heavy tablespoon 50

Margarine, 1 cup
  (2 ¼-lb. sticks) 1,615
  1 pat or square 50

Oils, cooking and
  salad—corn, cot-
  tonseed, olive,
  soybean, 1 tbsp. 125

Salad dressings—
  French, 1 tbsp.   110
  Mayonnaise, 1 tbsp. 110
  Mayonnaise-type,
    1 tbsp. 60
  Russian, 1 tbsp. 75

Yogurt, plain, 1 cup 120

BREADS AND GRAIN PRODUCTS

Bread, all types, av-
  erage slice, plain,
  toasted 60

Cereals, cooked, av-
  erage type, 1 cup 105
  Dry cereals, un-
    sweetened, av-
    erage, 1 oz. 110

Crackers, Graham,
  medium, each 28
  Rye wafers, 2″ x
    3½″, each 25
  Saltines, 2″ square,
    each 23

Macaroni, spaghetti,
  cooked, 1 cup 155

Muffins, 3″ size, av-
  erage, each 140

Noodles, egg, cooked,

1 cup 200

Pancakes, 4″, each .. 55

Rice, cooked, 1 cup .. 200

Rolls, medium size,
  average, each 130

Waffles, average size,
  each 240

DESSERTS, SWEETS

Cakes, Angel food,
    2″ sector 110
  Chocolate layer,
    2″ sector 420
  Cupcake, 2¾″, with
    icing, each 160
  Plain cake, 3″ x 2″
    x 1½″ piece 180
  Sponge cake, 2″
    sector 115

Candy, Caramels,
    fudge, 1 oz. 120
  Chocolate, milk or
    dark, 1 oz. 145

Cookies, Average
    type, 3″ round,
    each 110
  Fig bar, small, each 55

Chocolate syrup,
    1 tbsp. 20

Doughnuts, medium,
    plain, each 135

Gelatin dessert, ½ cup 80
    sugar-free 10

Honey, 1 tbsp. 60

Ice cream, ½ cup 200
  Ice cream soda,
    average size 350

Ice milk, 1 cup 285

Jams, jellies, pre-
serves, 1 tbsp. 55

Pies, apple, other
fruits, 4″ sector .. 330

Custard, pumpkin,
4″ sector 265

Lemon meringue,
4″ sector 300

Puddings, custard,
cornstarch, 1 cup 275

Sherbet, ices, ½ cup .. 120

Sugar, granulated,
1 tsp. 16

Sugar granulated,
1 cup 770

Syrup, 1 tbsp. 55

MISCELLANEOUS

Beverages, Coffee, tea,
plain 0

Beer, 8 oz. 110

Cocktail, average .. 150

Gin, Scotch, vodka,
whiskey, av-
erage, 1 oz. 75

Carbonated bever-
ages, ginger

ale, 8 oz. 80

Cola-type, 8 oz. 105

Cocoa, cup 235

Ketchup, chili sauce,
1 tbsp. 15

Olives, green and
ripe, large,
each, average 9

Nuts, Peanuts,
roasted, shelled,
½ cup 420

Peanut butter,
1 tbsp. 90

Cashews, pecans,
walnuts, ½ cup .. 375

Pickles, dill 4″, sweet
3″, each 18

Pizza, cheese, 6″
wedge 200

Soups, Bouillon,
broth, con-
somme, 1 cup 10

Chicken, tomato,
vegetable 80

Creamed, aspara-
gus, mushroom,
1 cup 200

Rice, noodle, bar-
ley, 1 cup 115

MAKE A GAME OF MAINTENANCE EATING

Your positive attitude is one of the most important elements in maintaining your slim figure once you attain it through Quick Weight Loss dieting. Instead of grumbling about calorie-counting, make a game of it, just as many people enjoy working out number games and puzzles. Your game challenge is to pattern the

most desirable eating you can figure out each day
within your personal calorie allowance. There are dozens of combinations you can work out, so enjoy arriving at the answer that will please you most each day.
After a week or two it will become almost second nature to you to know how much you can eat of what
foods.

Never overlook or delude yourself about "hidden"
calories. For example, if you add butter to your vegetables, you must add in the butter calories to your
total daily intake. It becomes very easy to cut out such
extra, self-pampering calories. I've had patients who
said they couldn't possibly even think at first of eating
a baked potato or vegetable unless drenched with butter. When they did give up the butter because of the
weight-producing calories on the Quick Weight Loss
Diet, they told me eventually that now they couldn't
stand the thought of "spoiling the delicious natural
flavor" of the good food with rich butter. This will undoubtedly happen with you if you give it a reasonable
trial.

8. MORE QUICK REDUCING
DIETS FOR VARIATION

Note this again for your quick slimming success: For speedy reducing and staying at ideal weight, in combination with Stay Slim Eating the Quick Weight Loss Diet has been used more effectively by more of my patients and others to whom I've recommended it than any other reducing diet.

A very small percentage of overweights in my practice wouldn't stay with the Quick Weight Loss Diet for one reason or another. Some didn't want to do without fruits and vegetables even for a week or two. Some had an aversion to drinking 8 glasses of water a day. Others couldn't explain why the diet was not right for them.

Since my goal has always been to reduce the overweight individual—to *get that fat off*—rather than to force a particular diet, I worked with each person to devise the diet that would take off weight most effectively and surely in each case. This has resulted in my compiling a variety of quick-reducing diets, some perhaps bizarre (but effective) listed here with my personal specifications.

I recommend the same to you, to shift your reducing methods if necessary from one to another listed here. If one quick-reducing diet is very difficult for you to follow, or seems to bring on undesirable symptoms—whether real or imaginary—choose another more to your liking from the many in this chapter.

The one all-important point is to get that fat off you before it impairs your health drastically and irreparably. Every extra pound is an extra threat according to proved, inescapable statistics. The more excess weight you carry, the less your chance of enjoying maximum vigor, health and attractiveness, and living out your full years.

It's unfortunate that many dietary advisers overlook the vital fact that persons are as different and individual as fingerprints. With that in mind I've worked out for you here the many diets that I've created over the years for my patients. I believe that among these you will find the one diet, or the right assortment of diets, that will take off weight rapidly and then keep it off for you as an individual. What has happened successfully for so many others can and should work for you.

The Quick Loss method and all the following quick reducing diets have reduced individuals where "balanced" dieting methods have failed. Some people have found it helpful to switch from one of the diets to another after a week or two, for variety. The choice is yours. Either the Quick Loss or the other diets here can be your most productive route to a slimmer, trimmer figure and a new dimension in vigorous, healthful living.

LOW-FAT OR "FAT-FREE" DIET

This low-fat or "fat-free" diet has one fundamental rule: fat in any form, visible or invisible, is eliminated. You have a wide choice of foods but you must not deviate.

Stay on this diet for months if necessary until you're at your desired weight. After you're down to ideal weight, you can start counting calories and add a little fat to your diet. Until then, no fats.

This has proved to be a successful diet for many patients. After a few weeks on this diet, the idea of eating any fatty foods usually becomes repugnant to the individual. He generally reduces his intake of fatty foods eagerly from then on, even when back on Stay Slim Eating.

Choose from the following foods, eat only enough to appease your hunger, then stop. It's better to eat when hungry, six times a day rather than three times a day, if practical for you. In any case, by restricting yourself to the low-fat "yes" foods here, you'll lose weight surely and steadily.

"YES" FOODS, YOUR CHOICE:

"NO" FOODS, DO NOT EAT:

Meats: Broiled, boiled or roasted beef, beef liver, lamb, veal, chicken, turkey—all with all visible fat removed.

NO bacon, bologna, frankfurters, ham, pork, salami, sausage. No smoked meats. No smoked poultry. No duck.

Fish and Seafood: Carp, cod, flounder, haddock, whitefish, white perch. Clams, crabmeat, lobster, mussels, oysters, scallops, shrimp.

NO salmon, sardines, tuna fish. No smoked or fried fish or seafood.

Vegetables: Canned, fresh or frozen asparagus, eggplant, green beans, lettuce, peas, potatoes (boiled, baked, mashed, no butter or margarine), spinach and all greens, all types of squash, string beans, tomatoes. (Gaseous vegetables on consent of doctor: broccoli, cabbage, cauliflower, corn, cucumbers, green peppers, radishes, turnips.)

NO artichoke, avocado, dried beans and peas, French fried potatoes, potato chips.

"YES" FOODS, YOUR CHOICE

"NO" FOODS, DO NOT EAT:

Fruits: All fruits and fruit juices—canned, fresh or frozen.

Dairy Products: Skim milk (fresh or dried), cultured buttermilk, cottage cheese, pot cheese, farmer cheese. 1 egg 3 times a week.

NO evaporated milk, whole milk, sweet or sour cream. No cheeses except those named in "yes" foods at left. No butter, margarine.

Breads and Cereals: Breads, rolls. Rice. Macaroni products—noodles, spaghetti. All cooked and dry cereals. Saltines, soda crackers.

NO egg noodles or fried noodles.

Desserts and Miscellaneous: Cornstarch, corn syrup. Honey. Jams, jellies. Gelatin, Tapioca. Ketchup, pickles, mustard, spices. Coffee, tea (no cream or whole milk). Plain sugar candy without chocolate or butter, moderately.

NO fried foods. No olive oil, vegetable oil, lard, suet, bacon fat. No olives, nuts, peanut butter. No mayonnaise, commercial salad dressings. No cakes, cookies, doughnuts, pastries, pies. No chocolate or cocoa.

Make up your meals from the preceding listing, checking the calorie counts from the listing in Chapter 7. For example, here's a typical day's menu. Eating moderate portions, you would consume 1,300 to 1,400 calories on this selection.

Breakfast	Lunch	Dinner
Fruit or fruit juice	Either lean meat or fish or cottage cheese, or poultry without skin	Either meat or fish or cottage cheese, or poultry without skin
Any one: Cereal with skim milk, or egg, or bread with jam or jelly Coffee or tea	Vegetable or salad	Vegetable or salad
	Any one: Potato or rice or noodles or bread with jam or jelly	Any one: Potato or rice or noodles or bread with jam or jelly
	Fruit or gelatin	Fruit or gelatin
	Coffee or tea	Coffee or tea

On this diet, you will lose between 2 and 5 pounds a week on an average, depending on how much you're overweight. You can take vitamin tablets to supplement the diet although this should not be needed. This is a relatively easy diet to stay on for months if necessary.

L-C L-F DIET (LOW CHOLESTEROL, LOW FAT)

This diet is not as low in fat as the preceding low-fat diet. It is low in cholesterol for those who are advised by the doctor to reduce cholesterol intake. Eat moderate portions and you'll find this an excellent reducing diet although not as quick reducing as the Quick Loss method.

A newspaper report stated, "The American Heart Association recommends that everybody cut down on fatty food intake. . . . this possibly could reduce the risk of heart attacks and strokes . . . based on 'evidence from many countries that suggests a relationship between the amount and type of fat consumed, the amount of cholesterol in the blood and the reported incidence of coronary artery disease.' "

"YES" FOODS, YOUR CHOICE:

"NO" FOODS, DO NOT EAT:

Meats: Use lean cuts only, trim off all fat. Broiled, boiled or roasted beef, lamb, chicken, turkey

NO animal fats. No "organ meats," no bacon, brains, duck, kidney, liver, pork, sausage, sweetbreads, veal

Fish and Seafood: Cod, flounder, haddock

NO bluefish, mackerel, salmon, shad, tuna fish, whitefish. No oysters, shrimp, snails

Vegetables, canned, fresh or frozen: All vegetables including asparagus, beets, carrots, celery, eggplant, lettuce, spinach and other greens, string beans, tomatoes, turnips

Fruits: All fruits—canned, fresh or frozen—and fruit juices

Dairy Products: Skim milk (fresh or dried). Pot cheese, cottage cheese, farmer cheese. Margarine

Desserts and Miscellaneous: Breads, cereals (cooked or dry). Rice, macaroni, noodles. Saltines, soda crackers. Vegetable oils. Jams, jellies, preserves. Egg whites in cooking. Cornstarch, corn syrup, honey. Gelatin. Tapioca. Coffee, tea (no cream or whole milk)

NO butter. No egg yolk. No cheeses except those named in "yes" list. No whole milk, evaporated milk, sour or sweet cream NO fried foods. No egg noodles. No bacon fat, lard or suet. No mayonnaise, commercial salad dressings. No cakes, cookies, doughnuts, pastry, pie. No chocolate or cocoa

Here's a sample day's menu, using moderate portions:

Breakfast	Lunch	Dinner
Fruit or fruit juice	Lean meat, poultry, fish or cottage cheese	Lean meat, poultry, fish or cottage cheese
Either cereal with skim milk, or bread with margarine or jam or jelly	Vegetables or salad Any one: Potato or rice or noodles or bread and margarine	Vegetables or salad Any one: Potato or rice or noodles or bread and margarine
Coffee or tea		
	Fruit or simple dessert from "yes" list	Fruit or simple dessert from "yes" list
	Skim milk, coffee or tea	Skim milk, coffee, or tea

Average weight loss on this diet ranges from 2 to 5 pounds weekly, depending on how overweight you are. You can stay on this diet indefinitely.

Figure Your Own Weight Loss on Low-Fat Diets

In reducing fat consumption alone, the average weight loss is about 3 pounds a week at the start. This figures out very simply: The average fat consumption per person daily is 155 grams. On the low-fat diet, fat consumption is cut to about 30 grams; that's 125 grams less fat consumption daily.

Since 1 gram of fat equals 9 calories, the saving of 125 grams of fat daily equals 1,125 fewer calories consumed per day, and 7,875 fewer calories per week. Since there are 3,500 to 3,700 such fat calories per pound, the loss is about 2 pounds per week plus at least 1 pound of water, equaling a total weight loss of about 3 pounds per week minimum.

This loss continues for about 4 weeks when the weight loss goes to about 2½ pounds per week, lessening to about 2 pounds a week after 3 months. After 6 months the loss will continue at a slightly lower rate. Thus you'll continue to lose weight as long as you stay on the low-fat diet. When you're at your desired weight, you may stabilize at that weight by adding some fat to your diet.

Actually many individuals lose as much as 5 pounds a week and even more on a low-fat diet since they're likely to reduce their total caloric intake further than just reduction in fats. This is a fairly easy diet to stay with for long range weight reduction.

FASTING AND SEMI-STARVATION DIETS

One of the quickest ways to lose excess weight is to cut out practically all solid food, but not water, for a limited period of time. Various fasting or semi-starvation methods have been used for centuries and are increasingly popular today in taking off burdensome weight in a hurry. A big help is that after 18 hours of no solid food you usually lose hunger pangs and the acute desire to eat.

If you wish to lose 2 to 7 pounds over a period of 2 to 3 days, *the simplest fasting diet is to go without any food at all, drink large quantities of water and non-caloric beverages all through your waking hours, and take 1 or 2 therapeutic vitamin-mineral tablets daily*. If you wish to continue on this fasting regimen, it should be done under the supervision of a physician.

Another variation of this simple fasting diet is to do it 1 or 2 days a week, every week, as long as you're overweight. The fact is that when you're on any diet in which you reduce your calorie intake, you're fasting to some extent. By doing without any solid food for

1 or 2 days a week you're concentrating the calorie reduction primarily for the first or second 24-hour periods.

Some people find this easier to do than to cut down on calories considerably every day of the week. I have an increasing number of patients who would rather fast for a few days then restrict their daily eating drastically. They find that the large weight loss is a stimulant that keeps them on the fasting diet of non-caloric liquids quite easily.

Curiously those who go without solid food for a day or two each week usually don't then consume excess quantities on the days when they're back to eating again. Rather, the body becomes satisfied with less, hunger pangs are delayed, and the desire to eat constantly tends to lessen and even disappear. It would be senseless and ineffectual to fast for 1 or 2 days, then consume double your usual amount of food on the following days. This rarely happens after fasting.

Under medical supervision many persons have stayed on fasting or semi-starvation diets for 8 to 26 days, although there are reports of individuals on fasting regimens lasting up to 117 days (note examples on other pages). These obese patients have lost approximately 20% of their original body weight, dropping from 250 to 200 pounds or from 200 to 160 pounds, for example. Some losses have been reported as 100 pounds and more, with overweights dropping from 280 to 180 pounds in a year or less.

It becomes obvious that there is little chance that fasting over 1 or 2 days, or even 5 days, will be harmful for the majority of overweights. It must be emphasized again that you should drink at least 8 to 10 glasses of water daily and take 1 or 2 vitamin-mineral tablets. Again I recommend the Quick Weight Loss Diet as a more desirable way to lose weight rapidly.

On fasting diets, you learn quickly that you can lose weight by not overeating. You have proof that your overweight is due to eating too much rather than to any metabolic imbalance which you may have used as an excuse.

Above all, fasting even for only a day or two proves to you that you have the willpower to lose weight. From there it's a much easier step to the Quick Loss method and then to Stay Slim Eating. Chances are excellent that you'll never permit yourself to become overweight again.

If you go on a fasting diet for a day or two or longer, it's a great help to do it with another person or several people. Each helps the other with inspiration and watchfulness to stay on the water and vitamins diet.

I permit my patients on this semi-starvation diet to drink as much as they wish of coffee and tea without milk, cream or sugar, and unlimited quantities of non-caloric carbonated drinks in all flavors. This is a most satisfying aid in staying away from any solid foods while getting some taste satisfaction.

ONE-TO-TWO-DAY FASTING DIET

Here is a summation of the simple fasting diet which usually takes off 3 to 5 pounds a day:

No solid food at all

At least 8 glasses of water daily, and as much more as you can drink

Coffee and tea without milk, cream or sugar (you may use non-caloric sweeteners to taste), as much as desired

Non-caloric carbonated beverages, all flavors, as much as wanted

1 or 2 therapeutic vitamin-mineral tablets daily

In summary, if you go beyond 2 to 3 days at a time on this diet, you should do it under medical supervision; others have done the latter up to 117 days without any harm. Those who have fasted for a long time are usually satisfied with small meals thereafter. Most have altered the rapidity of bodily chemical and metabolic action during the fasting period and generally change their eating habits permanently for lower weight and better health.

350-CAL. PILOT'S DIET

Another variation of a semi-starvation diet is used for "rapid weight reduction for air crews," cited by Dr. Paul W. Musgrove, Lt. Col., U.S.A.F., Medical Corps. He states, in part, in the magazine *Aerospace Medicine,* "Overweight has been the cause of aircraft incidents, accidents and even fatalities . . . the trouble with most [reducing] programs is that they are too slow." Instituting a 350-calorie drastic diet produced excellent results in bringing down weight fast for most of those on the program.

Here is my version of such a rapid weight reduction diet:

Breakfast: 1 hard-boiled egg (80 cals.) and 8 oz. skim milk (90)

Lunch: 3½ oz. tossed leafy salad with non-caloric dressing (12)

Dinner: 3 oz. lean meat (160) and 3½ oz. tossed leafy salad with non-caloric dressing (12)

At all meals and throughout the day, 8 or more glasses of water and as much as desired of coffee and tea without milk, cream or sugar, and non-caloric carbonated beverages. Take a therapeutic vitamin tablet daily.

Total daily calories: 354.

Weight losses on such a diet are 4 to 6 pounds the first 3 days, and generally rapid loss thereafter. It is interesting that, as Dr. Musgrove stated about his dieters, "Several discovered for the first time in their lives that milk and fresh leafy vegetables are tasty foods."

An important point to think about is that if over-weight is the cause of some "aircraft incidents, accidents and even fatalities," how many more accidents and injuries may be caused by overweights driving autos? There is clearly another safety factor in being at ideal weight instead of burdened by fat.

LETTUCE AND TOMATO SEMI-STARVATION DIET

A simple semi-starvation diet used in some hospitals is this: 2 ounces of lettuce and 2 ounces of tomatoes at lunch, and the same at dinner daily, 4 cups of black coffee or tea without milk, sugar or cream daily, 3 vitamin B complex tablets daily. At least 8 glasses of water daily.

This totals about 40 calories per day. Some patients receive mild medication to counteract acidosis. Blood chemistry and other aspects are checked occasionally.

It is reported that on this diet, continued as long as 26 days, patients lose about 20% of original body weight. Most tolerate it well both psychologically and physically. Some of the dieters noted that the rapid weight loss encouraged them greatly and gave them a quick lift in spirits and eagerness to continue. They had no great desire to go back to excessive eating. Quite the contrary, it seemed an excellent preparation for comparatively low calorie eating for the rest of their lives.

Another advantage of the lettuce and tomatoes fasting method is that it helps provide some bowel residue. Of course, with any diet, milk of magnesia, mineral oil or enemas may be used to help the bowel function if required.

It must be noted again that while this very re-stricted diet produced no reported harmful effects, it was and should be undertaken with medical supervision.

6-MEALS-A-DAY NIBBLER DIET

If it's practical for you to spread your eating over 6 meals a day instead of the usual "3 square meals," then this nibbler diet may be exactly what this doctor would order for you. A phenomenon of this diet is that whereas 900 to 1,000 calories is the usual number allowed on a calorie-counting diet, the nibbler diet allows you 1,200 to 1,800 calories a day and you still lose weight to the same degree as the lower number confined to 3 meals instead of 6.

Why this occurs is not known exactly from the scientific viewpoint. But it has been established that small, frequent meals deplete fat storage in the body and use the dissolved free fatty particles for quick energy. The nibbler diet prevents the letdown feeling that some persons experience when the time between meals runs too long.

For those with coronary disease, small meals tend to shrink the stomach and help prevent pressure on the heart. In animal experimentation hardening of the arteries was cut in half among frequent feeders as compared with large-meal eaters.

It's worth reviewing what happens in the system from a heavy meal. The blood vessels are flooded with emulsified fat which slows the blood and may deposit fat particles on the inner linings, leading to atherosclerosis; the after-meal fatty sludge may clog and choke some of the narrowed, fatty blood channels. This is less likely to occur with frequent small meals which also have special benefits for persons with a high cholesterol count and those who have diabetes.

In short, the 6-meals-a-day nibbler diet acts to increase the lean muscle mass and decrease the fat deposits. It is helpful in preventing diseased arteries, gallbladder ills, gastric or duodenal ulcers and potential diabetes.

The nibbler diet is usually quite easy and even

pleasurable for many overweights. When you're hungry you eat, but only enough to satisfy your hunger, not in excess to feed your appetite. The custom of a coffee break at home and at work has helped to prepare many people for the nibbler diet. The vital caution is that this break must consist *only* of coffee or tea and perhaps a little something extra, as in the diet that follows, but not a doughnut or other pastry.

To help change your eating habits from 3 sizable meals a day to 6 small meals a day, you might go on the 48-hour fasting diet described previously. This has proved helpful in breaking undesirable eating habits, leaving less desire for big meals.

A SAMPLE NIBBLER DIET

Breakfast: 1 slice toast, 2 tablespoons dietetic jam, 3 tablespoons cottage cheese, coffee or tea, no sugar but you may use skim milk and non-caloric sweeteners

10 A.M.: Coffee or tea, non-caloric sweetening, 1 ounce milk

12 noon: Lettuce and tomato sandwich, no butter or margarine, 1 slice American cheese, coffee or tea, non-caloric sweetening, skim milk

4 P.M.: Coffee or tea (non-caloric sweetening) or 1 glass skim milk, 1 medium-size cookie

7 P.M.: Cup of clear consomme, salad with low calorie dressing or a little oil and vinegar, 4 ounces of lean meat, poultry or fish, coffee or tea, non-caloric sweetening

10 P.M.: Fresh fruit, such as 1 apple or pear, 1 slice bread with dietetic jam, coffee or tea with non-caloric sweetening

This listing totals about 900 calories. You may add up to 300 calories of food from the calorie table in Chapter 7. You need not stay with just the foods listed in the preceding which is a sample selection. Choose the foods for your 6 meals to your own liking according to calorie counts in the calorie table, for a daily total of up to 1,200 calories.

Some days you may find that you have consumed from 1,250 to 1,500 calories. Don't be disturbed about occasional lapses. Cut back for a few days to about 900 calories, then maintain 900 to 1,200 calories daily. My women patients on the nibbler diet reduced with even 1,200 to 1,500 calories daily, and men on 1,200 to 1,800 calories. For desirable quick weight loss, start with 900 to 1,200 calories daily and then you may increase after you've learned control.

On the 6-meals-a-day nibbler diet, you will lose from 3 to 6 pounds a week depending on your amount of excess weight and size, and whether you hold your daily calorie count to 900 or allow yourself more. This is a successful form of healthful dieting that you can stay on for the rest of your life.

It's important that you don't fool yourself by eating one or more heavy meals and then having the 3 extra meals also. You must stay within the daily calorie totals permitted in order to lose weight.

Weigh yourself every morning. If, due to circumstances such as extensive entertaining, you have gained 3 pounds or more, go on a fasting diet for a day or two, or the Quick Weight Loss Diet for a few days to a week, or on one of the One-Dimensional diets. When you've taken off the excess 3 pounds or more, go back to the nibbler diet and stay with it. If you keep slipping off the diet, then switch to the Quick Loss Diet or another of those in this book to find the one that works best for you.

Unless you're one of the 5% who have some metabolic disturbance, you cannot fail to lose weight on the nibbler diet.

Important: The nibbler dieting technique of spreading the daily consumption of food over 6 meals instead of 3 meals may be applied effectively to any of the diets in this book. You will reduce more efficiently and swiftly by the 6-meal method no matter which diet you choose.

LOW-SALT DIETS

A low-salt diet reduces you in two ways. First, the selection provided is primarily from low-calorie foods. Second, the foods are so bland and there appears to be such a sameness in many foods that the dieter unconsciously cuts down on quantity and consumes less than 1,200 calories daily. Some may overindulge for the first few meals and then find that desire decreases. Because of the blandness of the foods, the appetite is curbed habitually. Most of my patients on this diet have lost weight steadily. They had no difficulty in maintaining ideal weight when they reached it. Some have lost 50 pounds or more, and then stayed slim.

Here is the listing for the low-salt diet that has proved effective for many individuals:

General rules: Don't deviate from the listing that follows, as with every diet here you must stay completely within the restrictions. Eat only enough at each meal to satisfy your hunger, then stop. No salt on the table; salt substitutes may be used. No salt used in cooking. No fried foods. No salted butter. Only salt-free bread. Only fresh vegetables, meat and fish—no canned or frozen. If Sucaryl is used, be sure the label reads *"calcium* cyclamate," not *"sodium* cyclamate."

"YES" FOODS, YOUR CHOICE:	"NO" FOODS, DO NOT EAT:
Meats: Beef, lamb, veal; chicken, turkey. Brains, heart, kidney, liver	NO salted, smoked, canned or pickled meat, no pork or bacon, no canned meat gravies

"YES" FOODS, YOUR CHOICE:	"NO" FOODS, DO NOT EAT:
Fish: Fresh cod, flounder, haddock, halibut, salmon	NO shellfish, no salted, smoked, canned or pickled fish, no canned fish gravies
Vegetables: Artichoke, asparagus, avocado, beets, carrots, eggplant, green beans, lettuce, fresh peas, potatoes, squash (all types), spinach and all greens, tomatoes. Also, broccoli, brussels sprouts, cabbage, cauliflower, corn, cucumbers, onions, peppers, radishes, turnips	NO canned or frozen vegetables or vegetable juices, no beans, celery, lentils or dried peas
Fruits: All fresh fruits and canned, cooked and frozen fruits, all fresh, canned and frozen fruit juices, no-salt fruit sauces (apple, cranberry, etc.)	
Dairy Products: Sweet butter, sweet or sour cream, cream cheese, pot, cottage, farmer cheese, milk, dry or evaporated skim milk	NO salt butter, no cheeses unless named in "yes" listing
Breads and Cereals: Salt-free only! Whole wheat and enriched cereals and bread, hot and cold salt-free cereals, salt-free rice, macaroni, noodles, spaghetti	NO breads or cereals that are not definitely salt-free
Desserts and Miscellaneous: Cornstarch, gela-	NO commercial cakes, cookies, puddings except

"YES" FOODS, YOUR CHOICE:	"NO" FOODS, DO NOT EAT:
tin, tapioca, olive and vegetable oils, unsalted nuts, jelly, honey, cocoa, coffee, tea. Flavorings: cinnamon, cloves, garlic, green peppers, lemon juice, mace, mushrooms, nutmeg, onion, paprika, vinegar	definitely salt-free, no commercial mayonnaise or salad dressings, no peanut butter, no salted nuts, no commercial ice cream, ices or sherbets. *No ketchup,* no mustard, spices or sauces unless in "yes" listing

Here's a sample day's menu, using moderate portions:

Breakfast	Lunch	Dinner
Fruit or fruit juice	4 oz. meat, fish or cheese	4 oz. meat, fish or cheese
Any one: cereal or egg or slice of bread with sweet butter	Any one: 1 slice bread with sweet butter, or rice or potatoes or noodles	Any one: 1 slice bread with sweet butter, or rice, potatoes or macaroni
Milk, coffee or tea	Vegetable or salad	Vegetable or salad
	Fruit or plain dessert	Fruit or plain dessert
	Milk, coffee or tea	Milk, coffee or tea

It's best to check portions of what you eat on the calorie table, and consume about 1,200 calories daily, as in the preceding sample day's diet. You may not lose much the first few days but then you will average weight loss of 2 to 6 pounds a week, depending on how much you're overweight. You can stay on this diet indefinitely but unless you should remain on low-salt intake for personal medical reasons, you can go on to normal Stay Slim Eating once you're at your desired or ideal weight.

LOW-SALT LOW-CHOLESTEROL DIET

This excellent variation of the low-salt diet also reduces the cholesterol intake for those who should avoid cholesterol. Follow the preceding Low-Salt diet but eliminate the following foods: No whole milk, no cream, no sweet or salt butter, no egg yolk. Lean meat and poultry only, all visible fat trimmed off, lean fish only. No cocoa. All the other foods in the Low-Fat "no" list should not be eaten.

ONE-DIMENSIONAL QUICK-LOSS BIZARRE DIETS

While most of my patients have succeeded in losing weight quickly and happily on my primary recommendation, the Quick Loss Diet, a small percentage have found that a one-dimensional diet was the best to get weight off in a hurry for them. On the bizarre one-dimensional diet where they were restricted to one food only, they were able to exercise their willpower best, give up all thought of temptation with any other food whatsoever, and lose weight rapidly.

Here are some of the bizarre diets which have proved effective. Some general rules must be followed. A therapeutic vitamin-mineral tablet should be taken daily as a safety measure even though it may not be necessary with some of the diets. Some of my patients have been on such bizarre diets for 2 weeks to 2 months without ill effects, but you should stop if you feel fatigued, lightheaded or disturbed. If you should feel faint, a little orange juice or a hard candy should be taken. After eating more for a day or two, you might try again if you're determined. No one with a health disorder should undertake these bizarre diets.

On the other hand, many patients who could not reduce any other way have found that they lost weight quickly and felt great after going on one or more of these bizarre diets. Some even followed one of the diets for a week, then went on another of the One-Dimensional diets, back to Stay Slim Eating, and have continued intermittently in this fashion.

Like some of my patients, you may read one of the bizarre diets, like it instantly and exclaim, "That's for me!"

On all the bizarre diets you may have as much as desired of coffee and tea without cream, milk or sugar, but with non-caloric sweeteners. You may take unlimited quantities of non-caloric carbonated beverages and calorie-free bouillon and consomme. Drink at least eight 10-ounce glasses of water daily.

On the average, those on the bizarre one-dimensional diets lose from 5 to 15 pounds a week, depending on amount of overweight and the size of the individual. The bizarre diets have proved safe and highly effective for many women and men within my experience.

I've had patients eat one hard-boiled egg daily for 2 weeks; 8 ounces of cottage cheese daily for 16 weeks; one chicken leg daily for 2 weeks, one 4-ounce hamburger daily for 4 weeks; one portion of broiled fish every other day for one month. In such cases it's absolutely essential to drink 8 to 10 glasses of water daily. For these individuals, with no serious illness or recent operation, no harm was done. Because of the drastic change of eating habits, a slight fatigue, headache or lightheadedness may develop. Such symptoms usually pass as the body adjusts itself. If they continue, a doctor should be consulted.

BUTTERMILK-ONLY DIET

This is a very simple diet, as are most of the One-Dimensional diets. 6 glasses of buttermilk daily, spaced out 1 glass every 3 hours. The only other foods permitted are coffee and tea without cream, milk or sugar, but with non-caloric sweeteners, also as much as you want of non-caloric sodas and calorie-free bouillon and consomme, along with a vitamin tablet daily.

COTTAGE CHEESE AND GRAPEFRUIT DIET

Moderate portions of cottage cheese and grapefruit —six times daily. Drink as much as you wish of artificially sweetened carbonated beverages, and coffee and tea with artificial sweetening, no cream or milk. If you prefer, you may substitute melon for the grapefruit, or alternate the fruits, using melon one day and grapefruit the next.

COTTAGE CHEESE AND BUTTERMILK DIET

For those heavies who are very fond of cottage cheese and buttermilk, restricting their eating to these two fine foods has proved effective and healthful in taking off 10 pounds and more in a hurry.

The diet consists merely of eating as much cottage cheese as wanted, and a glass of buttermilk, up to 6 times daily. This rarely adds up to more than 540 to 710 calories daily. Patients on this diet say that they find the foods filling and satisfying and they have no hunger pangs. When taken with vitamin tablets and large quantities of water and permitted non-caloric beverages, no deficiencies have developed in patients even over a period of months on this diet.

As with all one-dimensional diets, if you have an aversion to the principal foods, don't even begin! If you're going on a one-dimensional diet, choose the particular one that appeals personally to your taste.

BAKED POTATO AND BUTTERMILK DIET

1 baked potato daily, complete with skin, 6 glasses of buttermilk spaced out during the day. I've known some very heavy individuals to stay on this diet for months. As should be done in every such case, the blood and urine were checked particularly for any deficiencies. In practically every case I found the individuals in sound physical condition with health much improved by the sizable losses in weight.

EGGS AND TOMATOES DIET

This diet is a favorite among some of my veteran reducers who wanted to get off weight rapidly at the start. They continue to use this as a quick-action diet to take off quickly pounds which may have crept up on them. *They simply eat a hard-boiled egg and a small tomato up to 6 times a day, and only when they feel hungry.* The fat vanishes quickly day after day.

This and similar bizarre diets work amazingly for many heavy eaters because they undertake the one-dimensional diet as a challenge for a limited period. Thus they're able to wipe away any desire to eat just for the sheer enjoyment of packing in tasty food even when not hungry. Being acutely conscious of what they've set out to accomplish on the bizarre diet, they don't eat out of boredom or just for the pleasure of eating. I've seen some of the worst gluttons go on this Eggs and Tomatos diet, for instance, and stay with it. They lost dangerous and burdensome fat that they couldn't get off before.

MEAT ONLY DIET

This diet is limited to a half-pound of any meat wanted, 3 times a day, along with plenty of water and the other non-caloric drinks. For lots of those who like meat very much, this has proved an effective quick-reducing diet. A doctor I know of has used this as the prime reducing diet for many of his obese patients and those ill from excess weight. He claims that he finds this diet so successful and safe because "meat and water are the only two natural foods on this planet." One might question his statement but I can attest that a good many overweights drop excess fat rapidly with this meat only diet.

On this diet, eat lean meat, only when hungry and only enough to take away hunger. You'll lose great amounts of fat quickly, safely and surely.

POULTRY ONLY DIET

Follow the same instructions as in the preceding meat only diet but instead of meat, use chicken or turkey with the skin removed.

FISH ONLY DIET

This is another variation of the meat only diet; it has been used successfully by those who are very fond of fish and seafood. It affords a large choice from a wide variety in those categories. Simply follow the same instructions as the meat only diet but choose from any seafood and lean fish.

MEAT, POULTRY, FISH ONLY DIET

This diet affords you a combination of meat, poultry, fish and seafood during any one meal or confining one type to each meal. For example you might have broiled fish at breakfast, chicken at lunch, and lean meat at dinner. You might enjoy at dinner some shrimps, a small chicken leg and some lean meat. In general follow the instructions for the meat only diet.

ALL VEGETABLE DIET

Eat vegetables only, as much as you want of vegetables of your choice, up to 6 meals daily. This means exactly what it states—*vegetables only*—no nuts, butter, milk, eggs or cheese. Drink a good deal of water and unlimited quantities of the non-caloric liquids.

For many individuals, this can be a lifetime diet. If you're sold on it, can tolerate it, if no deficiencies show up in regular medical checkups, then you can feel assured that you'll never be heavy again if you become an all vegetable eater.

You may eat practically any vegetables outside of a few such as avocados, beans, lentils and sweet potatoes, choosing from this list.

	CALORIES		CALORIES
Asparagus, 1 cup (8 oz.)	35	Mushrooms, 1 cup	30
Beets, 1 cup	70	Onions, 1 cup cooked	80
Broccoli, 1 cup	45	Onions, 1 cup raw	50
Brussels sprouts, 1 cup	60	Parsley, 1 tbsp.	1
Cabbage, 1 cup cooked	40	Potato, 1 medium baked	105
raw	25	Radishes, 1 cup	25
Carrots, 1 cup	45	Sauerkraut, 1 cup	30
Cauliflower, 1 cup cooked	30	Squash (winter), 1 cup	95
Celery, 1 cup	20	String Beans, 1 cup	35
Corn, 1 small ear	65	Tomato, 1 medium fresh	30
Cucumber, 1 cup	20	juice, 1 cup	50
Horseradish, 1 tbsp.	25	Turnips, 1 cup	40
Lettuce, hard head	70		

If you ate most of the portions listed above in one day, totaling 16 cups of vegetables, plus 1 tomato, 1 good-sized head of lettuce and a medium-sized potato, you'd still be eating only about 900 calories. It's not likely you could eat all this in 1 day, so you can readily see that your calorie intake is small on an all vegetable diet.

You can make the foods more interesting with spices and a sprinkling of low-calorie dressing. You may vary the vegetables with fruits of comparable caloric value, referring to the calorie charts. If you stick to it, you'll take off weight steadily and you'll never be fat again.

The big danger on an all vegetable diet is if you start to relax and add vegetable oil dressings, bread, butter, cream cheese, eggs, nuts, milk and such. Before you know it, you add 500 to 1,000 extra calories per meal and up goes your weight. So, as with all restrictive diets, remember that there must be no deviations and no extras.

FRUIT ONLY DIET

If you love fruit, this diet may prove to be exactly what you want for rapid weight loss over the period of a week or two, as it has for others. Here's a sample day's diet:

> *Breakfast:* 1 orange whole or sliced, or 2 prunes, or ½ grapefruit
> *Lunch:* 1 small melon, or 1 large slice of a large melon plus 1 large slice of watermelon
> *4 P.M.:* 1 peach (or equivalent available fruit)
> *Dinner:* 1 pear, 1 orange, 1 apple, 1 plum
> *10 P.M.:* 1 apple

At each meal you may have coffee and tea without milk, cream or sugar. Throughout the day, drink as much as you wish of non-caloric carbonated beverages.

Your total intake on this diet will be only about 350 calories per day. If you really like fruit you'll enjoy the eating as you lose weight rapidly. Remember that this is a fruit only diet and therefore nothing else is permitted, no lettuce or salad dressing or anything else not listed in the preceding. You may substitute other available fresh fruits for those listed.

VEGETABLE AND FRUIT MIX DIET

This popular diet for those who like both fruit and vegetables is simply a combination of the two. Refer to the previously listed vegetable diet and fruit diet, mix the two, consulting the calorie table, and being certain that your daily intake doesn't exceed 900 calories. You'll find that you'll have to eat a lot to reach that calorie total. As with all these diets, eat only to satisfy your immediate hunger, do not stuff yourself beyond that point.

You may spread your vegetable and fruit consumption over 6 meals a day, as described in the Nibbler diet. Again, have all you want of coffee and tea without milk, cream or sugar, and of non-caloric carbonated beverages.

QUICK LOSS FRUIT AND VEGETABLE ALTERNATING DIET

This series of alternating quick loss diets works extremely well in reducing many patients who are considerably overweight and others who want to lose 10 to 20 pounds:

First week: Quick Weight Loss Diet
Second week: Fruit Only Diet
Third week: Quick Weight Loss Diet
Fourth week: All Vegetable Diet
Fifth week: Quick Weight Loss Diet
Sixth week: Vegetable and Fruit Mix Diet
Seventh week: Quick Weight Loss Diet
Eighth week: Fruit Only Diet

Continue rotation or alternate the weekly diets any way that suits you best. This system satisfies the desire of many for differing tastes so that each week's eating is looked forward to with anticipation. The change from no fruits and vegetables on the Quick Weight Loss Diet to an abundance of both is enjoyed, and the excess pounds keep coming off surely, swiftly, steadily.

Those who are not very overweight usually can shift to Stay Slim Eating after a few weeks. This specific alternating system can be adapted with many of the dozens of diets listed here. The choice is yours to attain that one essential goal: taking off weight rapidly and keeping it off for the balance of your lifetime.

SMALLER PORTIONS MINUS DIET

This simple diet depends on cutting down to smaller portions of the foods you eat normally, *minus* certain high-calorie items. Each portion for needed losses should be about one-third of the usual amount. This diet is easy to calculate but it requires a strong will to resist larger portions of the foods you enjoy and are accustomed to eating in greater quantity. A typical day's eating would work out as follows:

Usual Portions	Smaller Portions Minus
Breakfast:	
8 oz. orange juice 110 c.	3 oz. orange juice 40
2 fried eggs in butter 230	1 boiled egg 80
2 slices buttered toast 220	1 sl. toast, no butter 60
coffee with sugar, cream 65	black coffee 0

USUAL PORTIONS	SMALLER PORTIONS MINUS

Lunch:

6 oz. hamburger ..	360	2 oz. hamburger	120
buttered roll	180	no roll	
8 oz. peas with		3 oz. peas, no butter	40
butter	160	1 cookie	110
3 cookies	330	black coffee	0
coffee with sugar,			
cream	65		

Dinner:

martini	150	1 oz. whiskey	75
8 oz. chicken soup	80	8 oz. consomme	10
8 oz. steak with		3 oz. steak, no butter	180
butter	520	baked potato	
baked potato		no butter	105
with butter	205	8 oz. spinach,	
8 oz. spinach		no butter	45
with butter	95	half grapefruit	55
apple pie	330	black coffee	0
coffee with sugar,			
cream	65		

Total: 3,165	920

While most of the portions have been cut about one-third, some substitutions have been made, and "minus" items include butter, cream, sugar, pie. It may astonish you that the smaller portions minus method has eliminated 2,245 calories for the day. If the eater here were a man 5′ 10″ tall, his calorie intake for ideal weight would be about 2,000. On usual portions eating he would have consumed an excess of 1,165 calories to add to his fat. Or, with smaller-portions-minus, he'd eat 1,080 fewer calories than maintenance, helping to reduce his weight.

On a maintenance diet he could increase the size of his smaller portions to total about 2,000 calories and stay slim. If this kind of dieting appeals to you, and you have the willpower to keep from reaching for larger and extra portions, it's clear that you can cut down weight steadily this way.

You must keep in mind this difference from the usual suggestions of others merely to eat smaller portions in order to reduce: on my smaller portions diet you cut out completely those high calorie foods specified. I have found that this usually makes the difference between success and failure in this type of dieting.

BANANAS AND MILK DIET

If bananas are a favorite food of yours, and you like skim milk, this is a pretty well-rounded diet that will take off weight quite rapidly. A banana is 75–100 calories and a glass of skim milk is 90 calories. By considering a banana as one meal, and a glass of skim milk as another meal, and alternating them, you can eat 9 spaced-out "meals" a day and still total only 900 calories.

This is generally a filling, satisfying diet, involving no hunger pangs. You get plenty of protein as the milk contains 10 grams of protein per glass; each banana has 1 gram of protein also.

JUICES ONLY DIET

This juices only diet is a favorite among a good many Europeans for taking weight off in a week or so. The diet consists only of natural vegetable and fruit juices: eight 10-ounce glasses spaced out during the waking hours. No sugar is permitted, but it's fine to sweeten with non-caloric sweeteners. Remember, at least 8 glasses of water are also to be taken daily, plus as much as wanted of coffee and tea without milk, cream or sugar, and non-caloric carbonated beverages. Take a vitamin pill daily. Weight comes off rapidly. This is a good 2-week reducer, but may be extended for months without fear of protein deficiency.

SUIT YOURSELF ONE-DIMENSIONAL DIETS

Some of my patients concoct their own one-dimensional bizarre diets and have been very successful at taking off weight fast in a short time. To suit yourself, choose one or two favorite foods that are naturally large in bulk and low in calories. Figure out the quantity that will total less than 900 calories a day. Then space out the number of meals you can make from this quantity, supplementing as usual with plenty of water and the non-caloric liquids.

As one instance of a personal selection, a famous judge I know went on a one-dimensional watermelon diet during the summer. He lost 50 pounds and then went on Stay Slim Eating the rest of the year, never gaining back the 50 pounds during all those months.

YOGURT ONLY DIET

Quite a few patients have lost weight quickly and pleasantly on a yogurt only diet. For this diet take 120 calories of yogurt 5 to 6 times daily (total of 600–720 calories). You may vary the flavors as much as you please, keeping the total calories under 900 daily. Drink plenty of water and additional non-caloric liquids. If constipated, take milk of magnesia or enemas.

REPETITIOUS SAME MEAL DIET

Patients on this diet have told me that they follow it easily because all they have to remember is the food for 1 meal. They eat that same meal for breakfast, lunch and dinner, as follows:

- 1 slice of toast with dietetic jam or jelly
- 4 ounces of fruit or vegetable juice
- 3 tablespoons of cottage cheese

coffee or tea without milk, cream or sugar, as much as wanted, also non-caloric carbonated beverages

Each meal is about 170 calories. You may eat 5 meals spaced out (such as 8 A.M., 12 noon, 3 P.M., 6 P.M., 10 P.M.) for a daily total of 850 calories, or 3 meals for a total of only 510 calories. Your weight loss will be quicker on the 3-meal routine, of course, but even on 850 calories you should lose rapidly.

If you find cottage cheese more filling and satisfying than the juice, you may eliminate the juice and add 3 tablespoons of cottage cheese (total 6 tablespoons per meal); you'll consume the same low number of calories, resulting in rapid weight loss.

SKIPPER'S 1 MEAL A DAY DIET

Are you like the woman described in the following? She said, "I found I was gaining weight rapidly because no matter how much I ate during the day I had to eat a big meal with my husband at night. I went to my doctor who put me on a 'balanced diet' of a 'balanced' breakfast, lunch and dinner. But it didn't work for me. My husband insists on a good dinner at home or in a restaurant. I ate along with him and kept putting on weight. What can I do?"

It turned out that this woman didn't care for breakfast. At lunch she was at work and that meal wasn't important to her either. But she ate morning and noon because she was afraid to forsake "balanced eating." Her solution was simple: When she was convinced

that she wouldn't be harmed by drinking black coffee
for breakfast, then black coffee with a half of a grapefruit, an orange, apple or pear at lunch, then a good
dinner, she started losing weight.

Because she became accustomed to eating little
during the day, she found that she was contented with
less at dinner too. After six months she was at her
ideal weight and went back to the same doctor for a
checkup, telling him how she was eating. He examined her, then said, "You're eating 'crazy,' but your
blood pressure, blood count, electrocardiogram, are
just wonderful. Keep doing what you're doing, it's
good for you!"

I've checked many such patients with the same fine
results. If you're an individual who enjoys dinner but
doesn't care for breakfast or lunch, this 1 Meal A
Day skipper's diet may be just right to take off your
excess weight easily and pleasantly. Here's the skipper's diet that has worked well for many:

> *Breakfast:* coffee or tea, 4 oz. skim milk if desired,
>   and non-caloric sweetening, also a small glass of
>   tomato or orange juice if wanted
> *Lunch:* fruit (half grapefruit or an orange or apple)
>   and coffee or tea with milk and non-caloric sweet-
>   ening if desired
> *Dinner:* ½ pound lean meat (or caloric equivalent
>   in poultry or fish—see calorie table)
>   salad with low calorie dressing
>   half grapefruit or melon or 1 fresh fruit
>   black coffee or tea
> *2 hours later:* (if desired) coffee or tea and a piece
>   of fresh fruit; or a glass of skim milk with a
>   slice of toast and 1 tablespoon of cottage cheese
> *2 hours later:* (if desired) skim milk or yogurt or
>   a piece of fresh fruit; or coffee or tea with a slice
>   of thin toast and a thin slice of American cheese

The dinner totals 600 to 700 calories and the day's

eating 1,000 to 1,100 calories. Continue it—varying only the meat, poultry or fish—until you're at desired weight. Then increase to Stay Slim Eating as previously detailed.

Skipping meals is not recommended for those who tend to become fatigued, lightheaded or trembly. To find out whether such symptoms are real or imaginary, have your doctor take a blood sugar test at about 10 or 11 A.M. If your blood sugar is normal, the symptoms bear no relationship to lack of energy in your blood.

People who are free of any such symptoms can go on the skipper's diet for as long as necessary to reduce to normal. Once reduced, ladies, don't become so delighted with your new slimness that you continue to lose weight. This is not dangerous but is unnecessary and may produce listlessness. If you're a standard size 10 or 12, don't try to prove to your friends that you can get into a 9 or 7 dress, as some women do. This form of reaction is not found in men; they're usually content to become slim but not scrawny.

Beware on this diet of packing away a tremendous meal at night. This is especially dangerous to the arteries, which may become choked with fat, and taxing to the pancreas, sometimes leading to the production of diabetes.

To help curb any desire to eat too much at dinner, it helps greatly to fill yourself with liquid first. Before sitting down to dinner drink 1 to 3 glasses of water, or coffee or tea without milk, cream or sugar, or noncaloric beverages. You may not find this necessary after you're used to the skipper's routine. The excellent meal listed will slim you down and satisfy you too.

LIQUID AND OTHER FORMULA DIETS

The liquid and other formula diets packed in cans and other packages have been helpful to many people and may be effective for you in losing 2 to 5 pounds a week. Even the general medical profession has accepted the fact that they are not harmful to the average overweight, but have benefits for many.

It helps keep intelligent perspective to realize that formula diets are not new. Infants have been on formula diets for many years, or breast fed which is in effect a formula diet. The Rockefeller Institute had some individuals on liquid formula diets for as long as 4 years. Many doctors made up their own powdered foods for patients to mix with water or milk.

When the commercial formula dieting products became so popular a few years ago the first outcry from many doctors and nutritionists was *against*. They protested that this was drastic dieting at its worst! Then a more reasonable viewpoint took over. Dr. Vincent P. Dole stated in an editorial in the N.Y. State Medical Journal that, ". . . formula diets are not radically new. Physicians have used liquid diets in the treatment of disease since at least the time of Hippocrates, and more recently have employed nutrient mixtures for complete feeding of infants."

While emphasizing that "liquid mixtures do not have magic properties," Dr. Dole agreed that liquid dieting is not dangerous for it has the same nutrient qualities as any nutritive solid diet, and has the added factor of exact calculations not found in many low calorie diets.

If the liquid formula diet appeals to you individually more than the Quick Loss or other diets here, go on it with specific understanding. One advantage of the packaged diets is that if you wish to add 225 more calories a day, you simply take another portion. However, this is a highly disciplined, monotonous way of dieting. Be prepared to stay with it for at least 3 months to take off a lot of weight. Go at it gradually, not all-liquid at once, as I advise in the following liquid formula diet. If not, you may develop a slight diarrhea or a bloated feeling of discomfort which may cause you to drop the diet. The following will help you succeed, on a formula diet.

LIQUID FORMULA DIET

First 3 days—1 glass for breakfast, then 675 calories of varied regular foods divided into lunch, dinner and/or snacks (use calorie table to figure out calories) For example, choose from lean meat, poultry or fish, salad with low-calorie dressing, fresh fruit, low-calorie vegetables, etc.

4th to 6th days—1 glass for lunch, and 675 calories of varied foods for other meals

7th to 9th days—1 glass for dinner, and 675 calories of varied foods for other meals

10th day—1 glass for breakfast, 1 glass for lunch, 450 calories of varied foods for dinner

11th day—1 glass for breakfast, 1 glass for dinner, 450 calories of varied foods for lunch

12th day—1 glass for breakfast, 1 glass for lunch, 1 glass for snack, 225 calories of varied foods for dinner

13th day—1 glass for lunch, 1 glass for dinner, 1 glass for snack, 225 calories of varied food for breakfast

14th day—1 glass for breakfast, 1 glass for dinner, 1 glass for snack, 225 calories of varied foods for lunch

Thereafter—all-liquid formula diet, 4 glasses a day for breakfast, lunch, dinner, snack—total 900 calories

You may interchange 225-calorie formula portions of wafers or soups with the drink if you wish, at any time.

In addition to the formula, drink as much as you want of water (the more the better), coffee and tea without milk, cream or sugar, and non-caloric carbonated beverages.

FORMULA AND ALTERNATE DIETS

Some of my patients, because of their individual characteristics which may be like yours, have reduced

very happily by alternating a liquid formula diet with
other quick-action diets listed in this chapter. For example, you can go on the liquid formula diet for three
days or a week, then a few days on the cottage cheese
and fruit or all vegetable or all fruit or other diet of
your personal selection.

As long as you keep your dieting at 900 calories
or up to 1,200 calories or so a day, you're going to lose
weight, and that's the objective.

10-DAY FORMULA AND MEAT DIET

This bizarre diet which I worked out for some patients utilizes only the commercially prepared liquid
"formula foods" plus a meat dinner daily. It satisfies
many people more than a one-dimensional diet. Follow this diet every day, no variations permitted, and
you can lose weight quickly and quite pleasantly:

Breakfast: 1 glass of liquid formula
Lunch: 1 portion of formula soup or formula wafers
Dinner: 6 to 8 ounces of lean meat or poultry, mod-
    erate portion of a vegetable, moderate portion of
    fresh fruit or artificially sweetened fruit
    At all meals you are permitted coffee and tea
    without milk, cream or sugar, unlimited quantity
    of non-caloric beverages.

TEMPTATION DIETS

This "newly beautiful" patient, Mrs. A., had reduced
in a few months from 160 to 130 pounds. She still had
10 pounds to lose for her ideal weight of 120. Now
she said to me pathetically, "I'm thrilled about being
slim again, Doctor, but I'm dying for an ice cream
soda."

"Fine, treat yourself to an ice cream soda. In fact,
you can eat 3 ice cream sodas a day for the next 3
days."

She looked astonished, said, "You're joking."

"No. This is what I call a temptation diet. You yield to temptation. You eat the ice cream soda, or whatever particular calorie-rich item you crave. You eat it 3 times a day for 1 day or 3 days or even more. But that's just about all you eat, except for a few low-calorie foods to make up your daily total of 1,200 calories."

"Won't I pile on weight in a hurry?"

"No. You'll still be consuming less than your daily caloric requirements. Three ice cream sodas will total 1,050 calories, about 350 calories each, well below your daily requirement in respect to reducing."

Many doctors and nutritionists may deride this as a "screwball" dieting idea, but it works. I know it works because it has helped slim many hundreds of people within my experience, safely and effectively. By yielding to temptation this way, you satisfy any craving for the calorie-rich food. In fact, after you have 3 ice cream sodas in a day, for example, let alone for 3 days, you're so sick of ice cream sodas that you may never crave them again. And you realize that you really hadn't deprived yourself of anything wonderful, that there's much greater reward in being thin than in being a glutton.

What's your temptation, if any? Is it ice cream, pie a la mode, or just plenty of fresh bread and butter? Do you crave a sweet baked apple with cream, waffles or pancakes with butter and syrup?

Most dieters lose a craving after going on the Quick Weight Loss Diet, or one of the drastic bizarre diets. But if the craving is really strong, let yourself go. *However, keep your intake within your daily caloric allowance.* Don't add these temptation foods to the others; subtract them from the total.

Suppose your allowance for reducing is 1,200 calories a day. (Stay Slim Eating usually runs much higher.) If your temptation snacks, such as 2 ice cream sodas, total 700 calories, you have 500 calories left for

the balance of your day's eating. That means you can
eat, for example, plenty of certain vegetables, a sizable
portion of salad with low-calorie dressing, a boiled
egg, a thin slice of bread. And you can have all you
want of non-caloric bouillon, sugarless coffee, tea and
non-caloric beverages.

Do you crave pie a la mode? Have orange juice
and coffee for breakfast, pie a la mode and coffee or
tea for lunch, pie a la mode and coffee or tea for
dinner, snacks of non-caloric bouillon and non-caloric
carbonated beverages, as much as you want. You'll
still total only about 1,200 calories per day (and you
won't want to look at pie a la mode for quite a while).

Is such eating dangerous to health? Absolutely not
for a few days, a week, even a few weeks. Beyond
that, a doctor should check you for any abnormalities
in the blood or otherwise. As an extra measure, take
a vitamin tablet daily. Don't forget that many clinics
prescribe total abstinence from food for 7 to 14 days
and longer. Many patients, under supervision, have
had only orange juice and non-caloric liquids for 60
to 80 days, and taken off excess weight healthfully.

A woman complained to me, "All my husband eats
for breakfast is a scoop of ice cream and black coffee,
yet he stays thin and I get fat." I said, "Fine, the ice
cream has only as many calories as a dish of oatmeal.
He's having about 150 calories for breakfast, that's very
little." I added up the foods she was eating and found
that she was averaging an 800-calorie breakfast before she came to me. She reduced quickly with the
Quick Loss method.

I certainly don't advocate ice cream sodas and pie a
la mode and such as a permanent way of eating. Aside
from caloric content, such rich foods may affect an
acne condition or other skin problem, for example.
But, as instructed here, yield to temptation on the
temptation diet if it helps you to keep losing weight.
Like most of my patients who have done it, you'll find
that temptation soon gets behind thee.

DAY-IN DAY-OUT DIET

This simple "lopsided" diet has served to reduce many patients in a hurry. You stick to the same menu day-in day-out for weeks. The very one-dimensional monotonous aspect of the eating is its most effective feature. As on many restricted diets, you lose your desire for much food after a few days. Total calorie intake is only 600 on the following:

Breakfast: orange juice, black coffee without milk, cream or sugar

Lunch and Dinner: average portion of cottage cheese, a sliced tomato, 1 slice of bread, 1 teaspoon of jam
Coffee or tea—as much as wanted throughout the day, without milk, cream or sugar

Drink 6 to 8 glasses of water daily and unlimited quantities of non-caloric carbonated beverages. 1 therapeutic vitamin tablet daily. If hungry, add 1 glass of buttermilk daily for 685 calories total.

LOPSIDED EGG DIET

For heavyweights who love eggs and should take off weight quickly, this lopsided egg diet of only 450 calories has proved very effective:

Breakfast: orange juice, coffee without milk, cream or sugar

Lunch and Dinner: 2 eggs—soft-boiled, hard-boiled, poached or fried or scrambled in no-fat nonstick pan, 1 thin slice toast, coffee or tea, no milk, cream or sugar

If this is too difficult for you, add about 100 calories a day with a half-grapefruit (75 c.), or a glass of skim

milk (85), or melon (50–75), or a slice of toast with
dietetic jam (100–125), or choose personal favorites
of about 100 calories from the chart.

Drink lots of water and all the non-caloric carbonated beverages you want, and take a vitamin tablet
or two daily.

RICE DIETS

A rice diet is very simply made up predominantly of
boiled white rice. This is not rice in its truly natural
form since the shell or coating has been artificially
removed. The best rice to use on these diets is the
regular or extra long grain white rice, or par-cooked
or par-boiled or converted white rice—the latter are
all the same, but with different names. Pre-cooked rice
costs up to three times more per pound than regular
rice, has much of the flavor already cooked out of it
and is less firm in texture.

Rice diets were originally introduced as an effective
treatment for high blood pressure. They turned out to
be fine reducing diets. Even though patients were permitted 2,000 or more calories a day, their weight kept
going down, for two reasons. First, the rice diet has
practically no salt. Second, because of the monotony
of the food few people on the diet ate their full quota
daily.

Here is the simplest rice diet. It will take off weight
steadily and add years of life, particularly for those
with a tendency to high blood pressure. It is not
flavorful and takes an individual with considerable
willpower to stay with the diet week after week. In
all the rice diets, no salt is to be used in cooking the
rice or any other foods, nor may foods be salted at the
table.

In all the following rice diets, drink as much as
you want of water, coffee and tea without milk, cream
or sugar, and non-caloric carbonated beverages. NO

fried foods are permitted. Take 1 or 2 vitamin tablets daily, particularly on diets No. 1 and No. 2.

RICE DIET, NO. 1

Every meal: 8 ounces of fruit juice
3 ounces of any fruit
⅓ pound of rice

This is a great deal of rice and it need not all be eaten nor is it usually (as noted, few people consume all the rice calories permitted on the diet). This same amount of food may be spread over 6 or more meals a day if desired. Take a therapeutic vitamin tablet daily.

RICE AND VEGETABLES DIET, NO. 2

Every meal: 8 ounces of fruit juice
3 ounces of any fruit
Moderate portion of any vegetable
⅓ pound of rice

On this diet also you will lose weight steadily and consistently. Nothing is to be added to the diet. No salt or ketchup, just a little pepper or mustard or horseradish may be used, but always sparingly.

RICE, MEAT AND FISH DIET, NO. 3

Every meal: Add to Rice Diet No. 2, a moderate portion of thoroughly rinsed lean meat or any fresh water fish, with no salt used in preparation or in eating. No seasonings with any hidden salt content, no salt or ketchup, a little mustard or pepper or horseradish.

RICE VARIETY DIET, NO. 4

Include some rice at every meal, and eat as much as you want of these foods: fruits, vegetables, well-

washed lean meat, chicken and turkey, fresh water
fish, eggs, cottage cheese, unsalted matzos. *Nothing
else is permitted—no salt used in cooking or eating.*

All these rice diets are excellent for taking off excess weight steadily. For those who are overweight
and have hypertension (high blood pressure) these
are literally lifesaving diets. The fact that the diets
are especially good for an illness doesn't detract from
their effectiveness when used specifically for reducing.

If you are not a hypertensive, after you are near or at
your desired weight, you may add a little salt to the
foods if you wish to make a rice diet your maintenance way of eating. Patients of mine have done this
successfully and felt wonderfully healthy.

After losing all excess weight you may add in small
amounts: sugar, molasses, honey; unsalted butter or
margarine; jellies, jams and canned fruits which are
not salted; bread when baked with fresh yeast only;
white vinegar; spaghetti; peeled potatoes. Salt should
be used sparingly if at all. If you start gaining weight,
stop using the unsalted butter or margarine and substitute mineral oil for cooking and salad dressing (combined with white vinegar).

Always avoid: salted or smoked fish or meats—
ham, bacon, sausages, herring, etc.—pickles, ketchup,
chili sauce, all such foods that have salt added in their
preparation.

The average American consumes about 6 pounds of
salt per year, and has been called oversalted. The
rice diets, like many other drastic diets, eliminate
much salt and water from the body, bringing down
the weight.

All my patients on the rice diets lost weight, but
none became skinny or scrawny. Self-denial is involved
in staying on the rice diet particularly because the
lack of salt makes food quite tasteless and removes
the urge and desire to eat. None of my patients felt
hunger pangs—it would seem that hunger pangs are

associated with looking forward to a delicious meal! You may feel assured that on rice diets you will lose the strong desire to eat, and you'll lose plenty of pounds.

CHOOSE YOUR UNITS DIET

This quick-reducing method pleases some dieters who like to make up their own daily menus from a choice of the whole variety of foods. Each "unit" equals 100 calories of food, selected as you wish, from the calorie count listing in Chapter 7.

The fewer units you eat per day, the more swiftly you'll lose weight. For quick reducing I suggest a maximum of 10 units (1,000 calories) per day. On six units (600 calories) you'll lose pounds and inches even more rapidly.

Example of a 10 unit (1,000 calories) day:

Breakfast, two units:
    orange juice, one unit
    one egg, one unit
    coffee or tea, artificially sweetened
Lunch, three units:
    four-ounce hamburger, two-plus units
    tomatoes, under one unit
    coffee or tea, artificially sweetened
Dinner, five units:
    five shrimps, one-half unit
    baked or broiled fish, one-plus unit
    broccoli and carrots, one unit
    lettuce salad with lemon juice or vinegar, one unit
    melon, under one unit
    coffee or tea, artificially sweetened

Dieters have told me that playing the unit game adds a certain zest to reducing.

SIX FEEDINGS UNIT DIET

Using the unit system, you will lose weight quite rapidly on 12 units (1,200 calories) a day by spreading the units over six feedings instead of the usual three meals, as follows:

Breakfast—two units
Midmorning—one unit
Lunch—three units
Midafternoon—one unit
Dinner—four units
Midevening—one unit

As with all quick reducing diets, you may enjoy all you want of non-fat bouillon, coffee and tea (without sugar, cream or milk) and non-caloric beverages.

900 CALORIE CHOICE DIET

You will lose weight quite speedily if you stay within 900 calories a day on a varied diet. To help some of my patients do this I have saved them the trouble of consulting the long calorie listings by providing an abbreviated list (given here) under the name of the 900 calorie choice diet. Selected items and their caloric values are given for each meal. Following the listing is a sample day's eating such as you might choose for yourself.

Breakfast:
Fruits: apple 75 calories, cantaloupe 50–75, grapefruit 50–60, melon 50, 1 cup pitted cherries 70, peach 45–50, pear 95, 1 cup diced pineapple 75, two plums 60, 1 cup strawberries 55, tangerine 35, watermelon slice an inch thick and 10 inches long 60

Fruit juices: ¾ cup grapefruit juice 65, ½ cup grape

juice 85, ½ cup orange juice 55, ½ cup pineapple juice 60, ½ cup prune juice 85, one cup tomato juice 50

Bread: slice white 70, slice whole wheat 55, slice rye 55, one biscuit 130, slice gluten bread 50, slice corn bread 105

Cereals: average serving of most unsweetened cereals about 100

Jams and jellies: one teaspoon about 20, one teaspoon dietetic 3–5

One egg: poached, boiled, fried or scrambled in fat-free pan 75

Skim milk: one cup 90

Lunch and Dinner:

Meats, lean: quarter pound 225 calories

Fish, lean: six ounces about 200

Shrimps, clams, oysters: medium each about 10

Chicken and turkey: boneless, no skin, 6–8 ounces 225

Cottage cheese: 15 calories to a tablespoon, 135 calories to four ounces (Can substitute pot cheese or farmer cheese but no other cheese is recommended.)

Vegetables: about 50 calories per sizable portion of asparagus, broccoli, cabbage, cauliflower, celery, cucumber, eggplant, escarole, lettuce, okra, peppers, radishes, sauerkraut, spinach, string beans, tomatoes

Salad: about 50 calories per sizable portion dressed with lemon juice or vinegar

Starches: potato 95, ½ cup cooked rice 100, ½ cup noodles or spaghetti or macaroni 100, slice white bread 70 (no butter or sauces on any of these or on vegetables)

Now, from this condensed list, you know exactly what calorie value each item has and can make up your own daily menu such as this:

Breakfast: ½ cup orange juice 55, slice white toast 70,

jam 20, coffee or tea without sugar, milk or cream—
total 145 calories

Lunch: meat 225, vegetable 50, rice 100, fruit 60—total
435 calories

Dinner: cottage cheese 135, tossed salad 50, slice
bread 70, melon 50, coffee or tea without sugar,
milk or cream—total 305 calories

Total for the day: 885 calories

While you don't lose weight nearly as rapidly as on
the Quick Weight Loss Diet, unless you cut down
considerably below 900 calories per day, this type of
diet has one benefit. You start learning to figure your
caloric intake almost automatically which is a help
when you get down to your ideal weight and switch
to Stay Slim Eating.

HIGH-FAT HIGH-PROTEIN (HF-HP) DIETS

Various diets high in fat and protein have been
offered for some years. With this form of dieting the
appetite for most people is well satisfied. There is a
feeling of fullness and of eating a lot, with no accompanying "hunger pangs" (which are more often felt
in the dieter's mind than in his stomach). Thus the job
of dieting is made easier. However, for speedy reducing which I advocate strongly, my Quick Weight
Loss Diet and others in this book are far more effective.

Because they help some people to reduce I include
my versions of HF-HP diets which I have found to be
understood most readily and to work best in this
category. Success depends on adhering strictly to the
regulations; deviations may well result in no weight
loss. It is a fact that through the years such famed ex-
plorers as Wilhalmur Steffenson and Admiral Perry,
Eskimos, and the Indians of the Northwest Plains
lived primarily by this way of eating. They were able

to perform Herculean tasks and were rarely heavy.

Of course their bodies were exercised considerably in their daily energetic routines. This is an integral factor in all dieting since exercise helps to firm soft, unused muscles, helps prevent sagging and burns up some calories.

In the HF-HP diets you avoid eating carbohydrates (sugars, starches, celluloses) and you utilize the stored fat in your body. The usual basic restriction at its strongest may be summed up in one sentence: *Don't touch carbohydrates, sugar, salt, fruits, cereals, bread, rice, potatoes, alcohol.* Much food is permitted but there are also many prohibitions. Use of salt is highly restricted or not permitted at all.

HF-HP DIET NO. 1

Eat plenty of the following, three times a day if you wish:

Any non-smoked and non-salty fatty meats, chicken, turkey, duck, fish, seafood. Leave fat on meats and poultry, and add butter, margarine and oil as desired. Fry fish and seafood in heavy oils.

Eggs fried in butter, margarine or oil.

Cream cheese, cottage cheese, sour cream, heavy cream.

Don't use any salt.

Drink plenty of water, non-caloric beverages, artificially sweetened coffee and tea with cream if desired but no milk.

No snacks are permitted. Eat plenty at each meal, as much as you can without overeating.

No fruits, vegetables other than lettuce and tomatoes, no breads, spaghetti, macaroni products, rice, potatoes, cakes.

No pickled or canned meats or fish, no frankfurters, bologna, salami, smoked or salted ham or bacon (unsalted ham and bacon are permitted).

No alcoholic beverages, no beer, not even dry wines.
A sample day's eating from the foods allowed:

Breakfast:
    2 scrambled eggs fried in butter or margarine
    3 strips of unsalted bacon
    coffee with cream (not milk)

Lunch:
    6 oz. fish or seafood fried in oil
    sliced tomatoes with oil or mayonnaise
    coffee with cream

Dinner:
    8 oz. of fatty meat
    salad with plenty of oil or mayonnaise
    coffee with cream

Snack 10 P.M.:
    cheese, or chicken, or hard-boiled egg

Make up your own daily menus from the foods permitted, along the lines of this sample day's eating, on this and the following HF-HP diets.

HF-HP DIET NO. 2

This is the same as Diet No. 1 but you add a cup of any one of the following vegetables at lunch and dinner if you wish:

Asparagus	Celery	Radishes
Broccoli	Cucumber	String beans
Brussels sprouts	Eggplant	Tomatoes
Cabbage	Green pepper	
Cauliflower	Lettuce	

HF-HP DIET NO. 3

This is similar to Diet No. 2 but you may now add some of the following vegetables (1 cup at lunch and at dinner of any one) which contain carbohydrates in a higher percentage:

Beans, baked	Peas
Carrots	Potatoes
Corn	Potato chips
Onions	

HF-HP DIET NO. 4

This is the same as Diet No. 3 but here you may add:

Half-slice of protein bread three times daily.

Half grapefruit or a small orange each day.

GENERAL INSTRUCTIONS AND SUMMARY FOR HF-HP DIETS

Don't try to gorge yourself at the beginning of your dieting as the abundance of fatty foods may tend to make you nauseous.

You may eat as much fatty food as you wish within the restrictions of the varieties permitted. Eat to the limit of your capacity at each meal but if you overeat you are likely to feel ill.

No smoked or salted foods, but water-packed salmon and tuna are permitted.

Don't add salt to any foods. You may season with pepper, mustard and dry spices.

Eat as much protein as you wish but only from the foods permitted. The proteins will come from animal fats and pure oils primarily; proteins in carbohydrates are generally forbidden.

Drink 6 to 8 glasses of water daily to wash out acids and waste in your blood. Drink plenty of water before, during and after meals. Without enough water there may be a tendency to become listless and tired on this type of dieting.

In general you may use any type of oil or fat or butter on these diets. However it is desirable, for men especially, to use unsaturated fats or margarine containing a great deal of corn oil, safflower oil, soybean oil, or cottonseed oil.

If you have been advised that you have a high cholesterol, trim your meats of fat. Substitute plenty of margarine for frying, and instead of gravies.

There is very little residue from this type of dieting so don't expect the usual frequency of bowel movements. If you feel constipated take a mild laxative such as milk of magnesia.

The body uses your own or the eaten fats as fuel on HF-HP diets. The sugar normally produced by the liver is generally sufficient to supply quick energy as needed. By drinking plenty of water as advised, you should feel sufficient energy.

Test your urine with *acetest* (may be purchased at drugstores). A drop of urine on this white powder will turn purple if you are following the regulations correctly.

Exercise in the form that suits you best for 30 minutes continuously each day (before breakfast is a good time for a brisk walk, for example).

Don't sleep more than eight hours of each day.

Take a vitamin pill daily.

GRAPEFRUIT-PLUS DIET

This diet is satisfactory to many. It combines the restricted foods for extra efficiency in burning up accumulated fat. It provides plenty of food and is a relatively easy diet to maintain if you like grapefruit very much. It becomes most effective in weight drop after five days, then you will lose steadily and quite rapidly although not as fast as on the Quick Weight Loss Diet. Follow this menu daily, varying the meats and salads:

Breakfast:

half grapefruit or 4 oz. unsweetened grapefruit juice

2 eggs any style
2 slices bacon
coffee or tea

Lunch:
half grapefruit
meat, poultry, fish or seafood—moderate portion
salad, as much as you want with low-calorie dressing
　　or lemon juice or vinegar
coffee or tea

Dinner:
half grapefruit
meat, poultry, fish or seafood—moderate portion
salad, plenty with low-calorie dressing, lemon juice
　　or vinegar
coffee or tea

With this diet you may not eat anything between meals; at bedtime you may have four ounces of tomato juice or skim milk. No desserts or alcoholic beverages are permitted. Enjoy as much as you want of artificially sweetened carbonated beverages, also artificially sweetened coffee or tea without cream or milk.

TWO MEALS A DAY DIET

This is a highly restricted, simple diet which has proved very popular and successful with a number of my overweight patients. It is easy to remember and takes off a pound a day for the average overweight individual, and two to three pounds a day, day after day, for those who are very heavy.

The diet consists of two meals daily. Each meal is a repetition of the other, aside from your choices within each variety permitted. Eat only what is prescribed, nothing else. Since you have a wide choice within the restrictions, each meal can be enjoyed—especially as you see your weight on the scale dropping away every single day. Each meal consists of:

3½ oz. lean meat, poultry, fish or seafood
1 cup of a low-calorie vegetable
½ slice thin toast
1 apple or orange, small
coffee or tea with a tablespoonful of milk if desired,
    and non-caloric sweetener
no oil or butter

You may use non-caloric salad dressing, lemon juice
or vinegar.

Use salt and pepper in moderation.

The juice of one lemon is permitted for the entire
day, may be taken as lemonade made with artificial
sweetener.

No substitutes allowed on this listing.

The calorie intake on this diet is 250 per meal, 500
for the day.

Have your meals at whatever hour you wish, only
two meals per day. After a few days dieters find that
their weight keeps dropping steadily and rapidly.

Stay on this diet for 21 days, or stop it earlier if
you've reached your ideal weight. Then switch to Stay
Slim Eating for two weeks. If you still have not at-
tained your ideal weight, return to this two meals a
day diet for two more weeks. Continue the alternating schedule until you're at your ideal weight.
Then proceed with Stay Slim Eating. Repeat this cycle
in the future as often as may be necessary.

Do not expect the normal frequency of bowel movements while on this diet because of the lack of bulk
ingested. One movement every three or four days will
be normal, especially if you drink plenty of water
which is highly desirable (six to eight glasses a day).
You may use a mild laxative, milk of magnesia or a
glycerine suppository as an aid.

The results of this diet are extremely rewarding.
With my patients, notable results have included up-

surge of energy, loss of breathlessness, lessening of excessive perspiration, relief from high blood pressure, lowering of cholesterol, blood sugars and uric acid. In a number of cases irregular menses have become normal, sex desire increased and fertility improved.

Many undesirable signs and symptoms associated with overweight have improved considerably. I've had many patients drop over 30 pounds in three weeks on this diet with no ill effects and with a most gratifying improvement in health and an uplifting feeling of well-being.

ANTI-ACNE DIET

While this dieting method is designed especially to help relieve and control an acne condition (which it accomplishes with considerable success), it is also an effective quick reducing guide. While eating properly is not the cure-all for acne, it is an effective and usually essential part of helping to prevent or clear up the condition.

With the anti-acne diet you eat as much as you need to satisfy you, *not* stuffing yourself. Enjoy plenty of proteins—lean meat, poultry (with skin removed), lean fish and seafood. It is of prime importance *not* to eat certain foods, specifically the following:

No fats, not even those in butter, margarine, cream, whole milk and whole milk cheeses. You can however enjoy creamed cottage cheese, pot cheese, farmer cheese and other skim milk cheeses.

No chocolate or other candy containing sugar; no cocoa.

No fried or highly seasoned foods.

No mayonnaise or rich dressings.

No pies, rich cakes, pastries, icings.

No pizza or anything with a rich crust.

No sugar-content sodas or other sugary beverages.

No alcoholic beverages.

There's a great deal you can eat and drink with enjoyment. Drink plenty of sugar-free beverages, fruit juices without sugar added, artificially sweetened sodas, coffee, tea. In addition to all the delicious lean meats, poultry, fish and sea food (use lemon or vinegar instead of mayonnaise), enjoy fresh fruits and vegetables (no butter or creamy sauces—use lemon juice), artificially sweetened jelly, gelatin and other sugar-free desserts.

If you have an acne condition your skin is likely to show gratifying improvement on this diet, as your figure slims down. The Quick Weight Loss Diet is also helpful in helping to combat acne.

ANTI-GOUT DIET

This diet is a boon to those who are afflicted with gout or have a tendency to suffer from it. Of course with this ailment you will be guided by your doctor's overall instructions. This diet has been extremely helpful to my patients suffering with gout, and is offered subject to your physician's approval in respect to your own case.

People who suffer from gout usually have an excessive amount of uric acid in the blood. They are generally heavy and are apt to eat excessively, particularly of the wrong foods. On this diet, meats and other foods high in purines (uric-acid compounds) are permitted in very limited quantities; in some cases meats are not allowed at all. Choose your daily intake from this listing:

Skim milk—2 glasses daily.
Lean meat, poultry, fish, seafood—no more than 4 oz. daily. Avoid entirely sweetbreads, sardines, anchovies, salmon, tuna, smoked fish, liver, brain, kidney, meat extracts, all glandular foods.
1 egg daily.
Vegetables—green, yellow and leafy—substantial

portions without butter or sauces. Eat sparingly or avoid lentils, beans, peas, spinach.

Potato, rice, macaroni—small to moderate portions.

Fruits—half grapefruit, orange or other citrus fruit, twice daily.

Toast or bread—3 slices daily. Eat sparingly or avoid whole wheat bread, oatmeal, whole wheat or heavy cereals.

1 pat of margarine or butter daily, used as desired.

Desserts—no chocolate or nuts. Artificially sweetened gelatin and citrus fruits are permitted.

No salad dressings; vinegar or lemon juice are permitted.

No soups made with meat extracts.

No coffee, cocoa or alcoholic beverages.

Sample day's diet:

Breakfast: fruit or juice
  1 small portion light cereal with skim milk
  1 slice enriched white bread (toast)
  plenty of very weak tea, 1 tea bag to ½ quart of boiled water; drink at least 3 cups

Lunch: vegetable broth (no meat extracts) or 1 egg
  potato, rice or macaroni
  salad with vinegar dressing or lemon juice
  1 slice white bread and pat of butter or margarine
  1 glass skim milk

Dinner: vegetable broth (no meat extracts)
  3 to 4 oz. meat, chicken, fish or seafood
  potato, rice or macaroni
  salad with vinegar dressing or lemon juice
  1 slice white bread
  3 to 4 cups of weak tea

Drink plenty of water all day, at least 2 quarts. 1 glass of skim milk midevening. Drink as much seltzer and artificially sweetened beverages as desired.

With this Anti-Gout Diet you can still enjoy plenty of delicious, satisfying foods daily from the listing. For those who suffer from gout this method of eating will help provide relief as the pounds and inches slip away and general health and well-being improve. It must be repeated that eating is a vital part but only a part of overall anti-gout treatment.

ANTI-BLOAT DIET (Anti-Water Retention)

This diet is especially helpful for the overweight who feels not only heavy but also bloated much of the time. This reducing method promotes an acid condition which stimulates greater amounts of water (urine) excretion. It brings remarkable relief to bloated persons with swollen joints, fingers, feet and legs, particularly in the summer months. It also helps those with phlebitis or varicose veins.

Each day you can enjoy foods in the quantities specified in the following listing, making up your own meals accordingly:

8 oz. milk
two 4-oz. portions of lean meat, poultry, fish or seafood
1 egg
2 half-cups of vegetables; corn is permitted, asparagus especially recommended
1 medium-size potato
4 oz. of unsweetened orange juice
3 slices of toast
1 portion of cereal
cheese, moderate portion
fruits—cranberries, plums or prunes should be eaten daily; for quicker weight loss drop the toast and cereal daily and substitute artificially sweetened cranberries or prunes or fresh plums

ANTI-ALLERGY DIET

For some overweight patients who are subject to a variety of allergies, I have created these anti-allergy diets. Individuals lose weight rapidly on this routine and frequently obtain some relief from their allergies at the same time (of course the diets did not replace specific investigations of the basic causes of the allergies). It helped to keep these overweights reducing by providing A- and B-day diets. Follow A for three days, then B for three days. If allergies subside, alternate A and B by days, otherwise continue three-day cycles.

A-Day Diet:

> *Breakfast:*
> half grapefruit
> coffee or tea, artificially sweetened, no cream or milk

> *Lunch:*
> salad of 1 tomato, ¼ head lettuce, 5 asparagus tips, lightly dressed with vinegar or lemon or garlic
> cold lean lamb or beef—2 small slices
> 1 pear, medium size
> coffee or tea, artificially sweetened, no cream or milk

> *Dinner:*
> cup of clear broth
> lean lamb, beef or chicken—1 slice 4″ x 4″ x ¾″ thick
> spinach—½ cup
> carrots—⅔ cup
> large artichoke with vinegar and mineral oil dressing
> 1 peach, medium size
> coffee or tea, artificially sweetened, no cream or milk

B-Day Diet:

> *Breakfast:*
> half grapefruit
> 1 rye wafer

bacon, 3 slices, very lean and crisp
coffee or tea, artificially sweetened, no cream or
milk

Lunch:
same as on A-Day diet, but add 1 rye wafer

Dinner:
same as on A-Day diet, but add 1 medium size
potato
and add a cup of sugar-free or artificially sweetened pineapple instead of the peach

On both diets add a pill of vitamins and minerals
daily. You may have all the artificially sweetened carbonated beverages and soda you want. Drink plenty
of water daily.

Stay on this diet for four to six weeks, or stop earlier
if you reach your ideal weight. Then switch to Stay
Slim Eating for two weeks, or from then on if you're at
ideal weight. If necessary to reduce further, return to
the A-Day/B-Day schedule or go on the Quick Weight
Loss Diet.

Selective diets for specific ailments and conditions,
and for unhealthy, diseased or malfunctioning organs,
are generally advocated now. They have been helpful
in many cases. Such diets for various diseases or afflictions are given because scientifically, experimentally
or through results in practical experience, they have
helped relieve chemical deficiencies or excesses.

Foods that may cause or aggravate illness in some
specific instances are omitted or reduced in these diets.
In respect to the diseases mentioned here, applications
and usage of different foods have some relieving and
curative effects.

Since each human is a complicated piece of ma-
chinery, many factors may affect his well-being. Some
of the suggestions for the use of these general diets
are given simply to supplement your doctor's orders

which should be followed carefully. I have no intention at any point in this book to treat anyone's specific ailments, but to be of aid by explaining to you how your doctor's diet and other diets may be helpful.

ANTI-RHEUMATOID ARTHRITIS DIETING

Rheumatoid arthritis is a diffuse (not concentrated) chronic disease which affects the muscular and bony tissues especially around the joints. During the course of the disease there are usually periods of severe pains. These are due primarily to the retention of inflammatory fluids around the tissues and joints. Your doctor can help you counteract the pains of the condition and should be consulted periodically.

With my patients I recommend the intake of foods high in vitamin B complex, and those with an acid ash content low in sodium (salt) and low in carbohydrates. Eating this restricted type of food usually helps in decreasing the joint and muscle swellings. Some of the foods recommended:

Acid Ash Foods: cranberries, eggs, fish, meats, oysters, plums, prunes, refined rice
Low-Carbohydrate Foods: artichokes, asparagus, cabbage, cauliflower, cucumbers, lettuce, radishes, spinach, brussels sprouts, string beans, tomatoes
Low-Salt Foods: beans, cabbage, cranberries, grapefruit, grapes, lemons, plums, watermelon
High B-Complex Foods: whole wheat, wheat germ

Typical Day's Menu

Breakfast: 1 slice whole wheat bread toasted
1 poached egg
tea or coffee

Lunch: 4 oz. meat, chicken or fish, or 1 egg
½ cup refined rice
½ sliced tomato
tea or coffee

Dinner: vegetable soup
             2 oz. meat with ½ cup refined rice
             ½ grapefruit
             tea or coffee (plentiful)

In order to make up the high B-complex needs, use an all B vitamin capsule and sprinkle wheat germ over some of the food.

The daily menus can be varied as you wish from all the foods allowed. Eat only limited quantities that will bring you down to ideal weight and keep you there. Overweight is extremely undesirable with this affliction, as with most other illnesses.

RAW FOOD DIET

This diet was extremely popular in Europe at the end of the last century for the relief of rheumatic aches and pains. Excellent results were reported, especially in helping the overweight.

No cooked fruits or vegetables were allowed, only raw. The diet provided sufficient eggs and cheese so that there was minimal water retention.

In this dietary format, fruits and vegetables should be raw but it is permissible to liquefy them in a blender or by other means. While I cannot agree with the curative values claimed at the time of its peak popularity, there's little question that if the diet is followed, within the set limitations, there will be a constant weight loss down to ideal weight. There should also be relief from the severe pains and annoyances usually accompanying this affliction.

You can make up your own daily menus, from the specifications already given, for this type of eating.

Breakfast:
    raw fruit of your choice, unsqueezed
    1 poached egg

1 thin slice whole wheat bread
tea, coffee, water (plentiful)

Lunch:

1 or 2 cups of raw vegetables, cut up if desired
1 piece of raw fruit of your choice
1 to 3 breadsticks, salt-free
1 pat of unsalted butter
tea or coffee

Dinner:

2 eggs poached, boiled or hard-boiled (no fat)
moderate portion of cheese
piece of raw fruit
1 slice of toast with jelly

Snacks:

4 P.M. and 10 P.M.—raw fruit, or raw vegetables,
or a few unsalted bread sticks

In this anti-arthritis diet, as in any diet, always try to avoid foods to which you may be allergic or which generally produce uncomfortable gastric symptoms.

If this diet helps you feel better, as it does many of those afflicted, you may stay on the diet for six months, but always make sure that you take sufficient eggs and cheese along with the other recommended foods (with the approval of your physician, of course).

ANTI-OSTEOARTHRITIS DIETING

The Osteo type is usually a growing-old arthritis. It rarely cripples like rheumatoid arthritis but its accompanying aches and pains can make life miserable for the afflicted. Common symptoms are neck and shoulder pains, headache and neuralgia, severe backaches, pains in the pelvis, groaning pain in the knees and ankles. There is a tendency for the person to be "always tired."

If you have these symptoms and they are diagnosed as osteoarthritis, you will certainly be under the guidance of a physician and will follow his advice.

Overweight aggravates and hastens this condition rapidly, increasing the pains and suffering. Heavy patients in my care are instructed to take off excess weight quickly; reducing as fast as possible takes the extra load off the aching body, legs and joints.

Here is the regimen I recommend to my patients (instructions for the diets are given in preceding pages):

1. Start with one to two days on a fasting diet.
2. Then go on the Quick Weight Loss Diet.
3. Stay on the QWL Diet until down to ideal weight.
4. Keep weight down with Stay Slim Eating.

Invariably when the weight starts to come off, the aches and pains decrease. Great relief is usually obtained when the individual is at ideal weight and never allows the excess pounds to pile on again.

ANTI-KIDNEY STONE DIETING

Many excessively overweight individuals suffer from kidney stones. Some of the stones are dissolved relatively easily through diets and medicines. Visits to a doctor, and following his instructions to the letter, are mandatory.

The counteracting aim in treating all stone depositing is to reduce the tendency toward calcium deposits. If the condition calls for the urine to be acid (you will be guided by your physician, of course), avoidance of all milk and cheese is basic and essential. A combination of high acid ash foods and low calcium foods is necessary.

Those patients who have uric acid stones or gravel are usually given an eating regimen which is just the reverse. This involves intake of a minimal amount of protein (meats, etc.) and an alkaline ash diet.

To make certain that the diet results in urine that is either high alkaline or high acid (whichever is called for in the particular case) a frequent litmus paper test of the urine is essential. In these tests, a red litmus paper turns blue as an indication of alkaline urine. With blue litmus paper, if it turns red the indication is an acid urine. This simple testing is usually done three times daily to get the most dependable results and guidance.

It is significant that with patients afflicted with stones, common findings are overweight and the drinking of too little water.

For patients who have uric acid stones or gravel, a diet like the following is often recommended. This is an alkaline diet and a low-meat diet. Here is a typical day's menu under 900 calories, making it an effective reducing routine:

Breakfast:
> half-grapefruit or 1 sliced orange
> 1 egg
> 1 slice white toast and dietetic jelly
> tea or coffee and water (plentiful)

Lunch:
> 5 tablespoons cottage cheese
> 1 sliced tomato
> 1 slice white toast and dietetic jelly
> tea or coffee

Dinner:
> 4 oz. lean meat
> 1 cup of vegetable except spinach or brussels sprouts
> 1 slice pineapple
> 1 slice white toast

Snack:
> grapefruit or orange, midafternoon or midevening
> Drink plenty of water with meals, all day and evening.
> Be careful to avoid eating cranberries, plums, prunes, spinach, brussels sprouts.

Only vegetable soups (no beef stock) are permitted.

No alcohol is allowed.

These high-purine foods are omitted, the same as in treating gout: anchovies, cookies, herring, gravies, meat extracts, organ foods (brain, kidneys, liver, sweetbreads), sardines.

Not more than four to a maximum of six ounces of meat are allowed daily.

With this type of diet, as with most diets, drinking water "plentifully" means 6 to 12 glasses of water daily. This is in addition to any other beverages imbibed.

For patients who should have acid urine, the recommendation is for a diet low in calcium, low in phosphorus, high in acid ash. It is suggested that the dieter take a great deal of tea and coffee plus all the water he can drink; taking over 10 glasses of water a day is highly desirable.

This diet should be high in chicken, eggs, fish, meats. General eating should include canned and cooked fresh fruits, cranberries, plums, prunes.

Avoid grapefruit and oranges.

Omit carbonated beverages because they tend to be alkaline.

Omit all rye, wheat or whole grain breads. Plain processed enriched white bread is permitted.

Omit any ordinary or special whole grain cereals. Refined rice is permitted.

Very few desserts except fruits and gelatin are allowed.

A small amount of salad dressing made from eggs is permitted.

No milk.

No leafy green or yellow vegetables.

No nuts or yeast.

Here is a typical daily menu which may be selected according to personal liking from the permitted foods:

Breakfast:
    tomato juice
    1 egg
    1 slice white toast or portion of refined rice
    dietetic jelly
    tea or coffee
Lunch:
    4 oz. lean meat
    moderate portion noodles or spaghetti or maca-
        roni
    1 sliced tomato
    1 slice white bread with dietetic jelly
    tea or coffee
Dinner:
    2 oz. lean meat
    moderate portion of stewed tomatoes
    moderate portion of refined rice
    moderate portion cranberries
    cooked fresh peaches
    tea or coffee
Snack:
    plums, midafternoon or midevening

This type of dieting is low in calories and qualifies
as an effective quick-reducing regimen.

ANTI-HYPERHIDROSIS (SWEATING) DIETING

Hyperhidrosis (excessive sweating) can make a person miserable and should be quickly counteracted. It
occurs primarily in the excessively overweight individual (there may be other considerations too, of course).
The water (perspiration) almost pours from the very
heavy person under many conditions.

Every crevice in the body thus becomes moist and
macerated (tender, soft, pulpy). The most trouble-
prone areas are usually under the breasts, in the groin
and the insides of the thighs. This condition is a

source of almost constant suffering for the afflicted woman or man.

The first and basic course of action is to get that excessive weight off rapidly. My patients are given this regimen:

1. Start with a one or two day fasting diet.
2. Then go on the Quick Weight Loss Diet.
3. Stay on the QWL Diet until down to ideal weight, varying along the way with other quick-reducing diets if necessary.
4. When at ideal weight, stay that way permanently by Stay Slim Eating. Go back on the Quick Weight Loss Diet immediately if weight increases more than three pounds over ideal weight.

The individual afflicted with hyperhidrosis should switch to cool, light clothing. Powder all tender, affected areas frequently, powdering the entire body whenever convenient.

Once down to ideal weight, and well launched on Stay Slim Eating, the condition usually vanishes.

ANTI-SKIN-TROUBLES DIETING

For any kind of skin trouble it is vital to consult a dermatologist before the condition becomes worse. With excessive weight the skin generally is more vulnerable to excess perspiration with its attendant problems of oiliness, inflammation, chafing, prickly heat and fungus infection. Again it's highly desirable to get those excess pounds off quickly.

It has been found that in many cases excessive fatty acids in the skin and in the blood predisposes the individual to certain types of growths on the skin and eyelids. These solid reddish and brown papules (swellings, pimples) may also be found over the body (the lesions around the eyes are usually known as chloasmas). A diet low in fat, and especially low in cholesterol, followed over a long period of time may help relieve and clear up this condition to some extent, if not entirely.

Follow the diets previously given in this book, particularly the diets which allow only a minimal amount of cholesterol and fatty acids. The diets attack the primary cause for a good many people by bringing down weight and alleviating skin problems perhaps due to the excess body fat.

ANTI-PSORIASIS DIETING

Those persons who are afflicted know too well what psoriasis is—a chronic condition involving erythematous (red) patches generally, which are usually covered by whitish scales. It may take different forms in individual cases. A physician and dermatologist should be consulted and instructions followed to the letter.

While there is no known cure at this time for psoriasis, many doctors believe that the condition generally involves excessive oiliness of the skin and in the blood. A diet which is very low in fat, fatty acids, triglycerides and cholesterol is often helpful to the afflicted.

Psoriasis is often associated with other fat disturbances such as oily seborrhea (dandruff), gallstones, osteoarthritis, and overweight.

Reduction of weight is essential as one step in combating psoriasis. The low-fat diets given in preceding pages are usually recommended and are often very helpful in obtaining some relief.

ANTI-DYSPNEA (SHORTNESS OF BREATH) DIETING

Dyspnea is the medical term for difficult or labored breathing, commonly described as shortness of breath. At the first sign of any such difficulty, which may derive from a variety of causes, the afflicted individual should see a physician and be guided by him.

With most patients in my care, I find that the Quick Weight Loss Diet is especially helpful when excessive weight is involved, and it often is. It not only reduces the overweight person quickly, but it also helps to draw excessive water out of the tissues and blood.

After getting down to ideal weight on the QWL Diet, the individual has the benefits of a smaller liver, a smaller stomach, reduction of fat around the heart, reduction of fat over the entire chest wall and reduction of the blood circulation through the lungs. All these changes tend to lessen the breathing problem. Shortness of breath due to excessive fat (or other factors) is a cruel affliction.

This is the course I recommend to my overweight dyspneic patients:

1. Start the Quick Weight Loss Diet *at once.*
2. Stay with this diet faithfully until down to ideal weight.
3. Then go on Stay Slim Eating for the rest of your life.

Patients who follow this routine find a wonderful new freedom in breathing and healthier living. They rarely suffer again from such difficult, labored breathing.

ANTI-ACID DIET AND ANTI-ULCER DIET

When the stomach secretes too much hydrochloric acid, it produces an hyperacidity which in turn results in heartburn, sour taste, a bloated feeling, and even pain in the pit of the stomach. In this condition, most of the spices, condiments and herbs which tend to inflame the gastric mucosa should be avoided.

All stimulants should be reduced, including alcoholic drinks, beer, tea, coffee, cola drinks, even aspirin products. Foods with concentrated extracts also generally irritate the stomach.

An ulcer of the stomach may be involved. This is an

aggravated, inflamed mucous membrane. Other factors such as heredity may enter into a tendency toward a stomach ulcer. Primarily it involves a very circumscribed small area which ulcerates and becomes very painful. Immediate and continuing physician's care is essential with such a condition.

It is helpful to eat only bland foods, without spices. The stomach juices must be neutralized. This requires eating often. There are two generally accepted eating routines which I recommend to many of my patients with this condition:

1. Drink skim milk every two hours, with a little refined rice or a few bland crackers.

2. Go on the Quick Weight Loss Diet at once, spreading eating out over the day, with only a few mouthfuls eaten every one and a half to two hours.

My patients who follow either form of dieting until relieved do not gain any weight. In most cases they lose weight rapidly when overweight, which is a great help in itself for the general improved physical condition.

Once an individual develops hyperacidity, whether from the type of food eaten or the large quantities ingested, he is almost always subject to recurrences unless correction is undertaken quickly and maintained. Persons in my care invariably remain free from recurrences by following the QWL Diet until down to ideal weight, and continuing to stay at that plateau. They are then likely to maintain good health, free from pain and discomfort; the same is true with any sensible, bland, soft, low-calorie way of eating.

ANTI-PROCTITUS DIETING

Proctitis is the medical term for an inflammation of the lower bowel and anal region. There are many local and systemic causes which your physician will investigate and treat accordingly.

Usually eating too much of highly spiced foods and drinking too much alcohol are involved. In the lists of diets given here, the Quick Weight Loss Diet or any of the bland diets provided will usually relieve this problem in a few days unless some special condition is involved.

It is vital here again that the afflicted individual get down to ideal weight and then maintain that status. For this purpose the Quick Weight Loss Diet is recommended primarily, followed later by Stay Slim Eating.

DIVERSION DIET

Occasionally a patient who has been reducing rapidly and steadily on the Quick Weight Loss Diet will come to me and say, "Doctor, I'm dying for something creamy. I must have something rich, not sweet but rich and creamy. What can I do?".

I have just the diet for this situation. I tell the patient to go on my diversion diet which I developed especially to satisfy that urge to eat "something creamy, not sweet but rich and creamy." I suggest that the overweight person eat nothing but the following for the next two or three days:

5 tablespoons of cottage cheese mixed with 1½ tablespoons of sour cream.

Eat this dishful six times a day at whatever hours you wish.

Also, you may have a cupful of chicken or beef bouillon (no fat), hot or cold, with each meal.

In addition, you may have as much as you wish of tea and coffee, hot or iced, artificially sweetened if desired, but without milk or cream.

Enjoy unlimited quantities of artificially sweetened carbonated beverages each day.

In case after case the patient finds that the diversion diet hits the spot, is "just what the doctor ordered." It satisfies the craving. The individual keeps losing weight rapidly each day. The reason is that the cottage cheese and sour cream mixture totals 110 calories per meal, only about 660 calories per day.

After two or three days the overweight has satisfied that particular craving thoroughly (or may stay on the diet a few days longer if desired). It usually meets the need for, as one woman said, "It is something that tastes like 2,500 calories but only adds up to about 700."

He or she is then ready to go back on the Quick Weight Loss Diet with its plentiful variety of good foods and the swift and gratifying drop each day of the numbers on the scale.

BREAD-CHEESE-WINE DIET

This diet has proved successful with certain patients who like wine and cheese very much and don't wish to give up alcoholic beverages completely while taking off excess weight rapidly. Extended over a period of weeks the diet has worked out well in such cases. The only variety is in the wide choice of cheeses and wines. Only light wines should be used, not the heavier types such as sherry and port.

You might wish to try this unique method of dieting for a week, then switch to the Quick Weight Loss Diet which permits you a greater variety of foods yet takes off pounds and inches most efficiently. Your goal is to take off excess, burdensome weight, and if you miss wine very much, this may be just the diet that works best for you for a period of a few weeks at a time.

Breakfast:
1 slice toast
4 oz. cheese (your choice)
coffee or tea, artificially sweetened, no cream or milk

Lunch:
   1 slice rye bread (or your choice)
   2 oz. cheese, your choice such as ½ oz. Roquefort,
      ½ oz. Camembert, ½ oz. Swiss, ½ oz. Cheddar
   2 oz. wine (your choice of light wines)
   coffee or tea, artificially sweetened, no cream or
      milk

Dinner:
   same as lunch

The preceding is recommended for rapid reducing.
If desired, add one half slice of bread and 2 oz. wine
as a midafternoon or midevening snack, but weight
loss won't be as quick.

THREE WEEK 555 DIET

This stringent diet has worked well for some individuals who have great determination to lose weight
fast and can stick to a rigid routine for three weeks.
This is called the three-week 555 diet because the
daily calorie allotment totals about 555:

Breakfast:
   4 oz. orange juice or tomato juice
   coffee or tea, artificially sweetened, no cream or
      milk

Midmorning:
   1 glass skim milk

Lunch:
   lettuce, large portion with salt, lemon juice or
      vinegar
   1 egg (any way, no butter)
   coffee or tea, artificially sweetened, no cream or
      milk

Midafternoon:
   1 medium-size apple

Dinner:

    large salad with half-and-half vinegar and low
        calorie dressing
    ½ slice thin toast
    cup of bouillon
    3 oz. lean meat or chicken without skin
    coffee or tea, artificially sweetened, no cream or
        milk

Have a vitamin-mineral pill daily. As much artificially sweetened carbonated beverages as you want. Drink plenty of water daily.

After three weeks, or if ideal weight is reached earlier, switch to Stay Slim Eating for a few weeks. Then, for further reducing, return to the three-week 555 diet or go on the Quick Weight Loss Diet.

The Quick-Loss diet is my prime recommendation as the fastest, surest, most desirable quick-reducing method for the great majority of overweights.

TAKE YOUR CHOICE . . . OR CHOICES

Certainly from the Quick Weight Loss Diet and over 60 other quick-reducing diets here you'll find one or more just right for you. If you reach the point where you can't stay on your selected diet, switch to another. For example, after a week or more on one diet, if you have a yearning for vegetables and fruit, go on the vegetable and fruit mix diet. If you want meats, go on the meat only diet. They'll all keep bringing down your weight.

Once you start on a stringent bizarre diet, you may be amazed as I have been so often, at the depth of willpower we humans possess. I've had a patient choose to eat nothing but ¼ pound of meat with lots of sauerkraut daily for weeks. Others chose as their personal rigorous diets raw chopmeat only, ½ pound of cottage cheese mixed with ketchup daily for 14 weeks, 1 hard-boiled egg every third day for 2 weeks.

These determined dieters lost a great deal of weight, felt well and vigorous. My checkups showed them to be in good health. I'm not suggesting such harsh diets to you. I cite them as examples of what individuals will and can do to get down to desired weight once they're sufficiently motivated. You can certainly accomplish needed weight loss for yourself through your choice of the many quick-reducing diets here that are much easier to follow than a single-food routine.

In following many of the bizarre diets, here are a few essential guides:

1. Quick-reducing diets are not recommended here for growing children (although I have treated hundreds of overweight youngsters effectively by rigorous dieting), or for adults with specific ailments such as diabetes or kidney, liver or heart disease. Such persons should be under the care of a physician, of course, who will attend to their reducing as well as other matters. These diets are not intended primarily to cure specific illnesses, particularly critical and serious ailments, but some may well be adapted with good results under a doctor's care, as I have done. They are planned to take off excess weight rapidly and benefit your health accordingly.

2. Most quick reducing diets limit your choice and intake of foods and therefore it is desirable that you take a general once-daily vitamin and mineral tablet. If you're over 40, take a once-daily "therapeutic" vitamin tablet. Calcium pills may also be taken if a calcium deficiency exists.

3. These diets are for a limited time, to take off the overweight which most persons cannot lose by "balanced dieting." After most of the excess weight is off, you start counting calories and go on Stay Slim Eating of foods of your choice totaling 1,300–2,300 calories daily for women and 1,700–2,500 for men (see Chapter 7). However, I've had patients on the Quick Loss, fat-free and other diets for a year or more. Vegetable and fruit diets can be continued indefinitely.

4. Since a quick reducing diet is, in effect, a deficiency routine, it is best to be checked by a doctor at the start and again periodically, particularly if you feel any ill effects whatsoever from the dieting.

5. You must stick to your restricted diet rigidly. No deviations or extras are permitted. By being faithful to your diet, your weight loss is swift, sure and steady. Drink a great deal of water and as much coffee and tea without cream, milk or sugar, also as large a quantity of non-caloric carbonated beverages, as you wish.

6. As explained in detail earlier, in respect to the Quick Loss method, when you reach your ideal weight and attractive figure, combine Stay Slim Eating with any of these quick action diets. Thus they can serve you not only in taking off excess weight rapidly right now but also in staying fit for the rest of your life.

9. CLEARING AWAY FALSE FEARS ABOUT QUICK REDUCING DIETS

Many persons have been blocked from dieting successfully by a fear that quick action dieting results in sudden weight loss that may be harmful. Another common concern is that the drop in weight may be followed by a gain when the diet is over. So they wail, "What's the use?" Furthermore they're afraid that such dieting may result in a seesaw pattern of successive weight losses and gains which in their minds is injurious.

The fear that this may be bad for an individual's health has been fostered by many nutritionists, doctors and other professionals, as well as by health faddists and others, who say that "balanced eating" is the only right way to lose weight. *I have never seen or been given any proof that this is true—although I have openly challenged this concept for years.*

I have accumulated clear proof in successfully reducing thousands of men and women that "balanced dieting" doesn't work with many people who are most in need of taking off dangerous, crushing excess weight. I have found without exception that with the patient who has no medical disorder the quick reducing diets I employ are safe and also are remarkably effective in a high percentage of cases. Nevertheless, certain prejudices held by doctors and the public die hard. Millions of overweights die earlier because of this.

As only one example of such prejudice, the accepted medical procedure after childbirth not long ago was to keep the mother in bed in the hospital for 14 to 18 days. Many doctors warned that cutting short this rest would result in impairment of future health for many new mothers. Today the new mother is permitted to walk about from a few hours to a day after delivery and to go home in a few days. Far from resulting in catastrophes, this change has speeded recovery to healthful, desirable activity.

Is restricted eating harmful or otherwise? Consider the case of U.S. Senator Margaret Chase Smith. A newspaper report stated that "Mrs. Smith looks less than her 66 years. Trim as a model . . . she usually starts her day at 6 A.M. and seldom gets home before 8:30 P.M." Does she stuff herself with a variety of foods to produce the necessary energy? No. "She lunches on powdered milk and cereal at her desk."

Two Miss Americas have stated that they kept slim, healthy and vigorous with very limited diets. When she became Miss America, Jacqueline Mayer said in an interview that she weighed 150 pounds at 15. She took off the excess weight by skipping lunch, going without breakfast and not stuffing herself at dinner. She radiated health and beauty on this bizarre eating routine.

No diet here is a fraction as severe as that endured by Helen Klaben and Ralph Flores when their plane crashed in the Yukon wilderness in 1963. In the first week they finished their "unbalanced diet" of tuna fish, sardines, canned fruit salad and other odds and ends that usually would be consumed in a few days. Then they had "only toothpaste and melted snow as nourishment."

Aside from the lack of food, they endured terrible hardships, temperatures to less than 45 degrees below zero, frostbite, gangrene, a broken jaw, broken ribs. They had no special protective equipment, no blankets or bedding. Yet neither one apparently suffered any lasting organic damage from their enforced fasting during the next 42 days.

I certainly don't recommend that awful experience in order to lose weight. But I've pointed out this example to many people who told me fearfully, "I'm afraid I'll damage my health unless I eat a 'balanced diet,' even if I follow a quick-reducing diet for only short periods." You'll learn otherwise, just as the airplane victims did.

In another case, one with which I was closely concerned, a young man of 19 left for service in Africa where he immediately had to change his eating habits and cut down his food intake sharply. When he was checked by his family doctor before going, his health was noted as only fair, with some rather serious reservations.

During his year working for a medical service in the primitive country, his diet judged by American nutritional standards could hardly have been more unbalanced and inadequate. He could rarely get any meat, green vegetables, fruit, milk, eggs, or many of the common foods available at home and in his university dining room. Like the people of the country, he lived mostly on dishes made with "mealies," tough Indian corn which is the staple food there, but is fed to cattle and pigs here. Very often he had to skip meals completely because there wasn't enough food around. In the remote mountains he went without sufficient food for weeks, gorging occasionally on meat when an animal was killed. In effect he lived on a semi-starvation diet.

He returned after the year without having had any illness while away. When his doctor examined him again, he found the boy a few pounds underweight but in better physical condition than when he had departed. The doctor commented, "Maybe I should put many patients on semi-starvation diets with hard labor for a year."

Compare the good sense of Quick Loss dieting with the operation of a good machine. Any mechanic will tell you that if you run the average machine at a nor-

mal working pace (ideal weight) day after day, you
have the best chance of getting maximum service
from it, without breakdowns. This kind of moderate
operating pattern will usually insure longest working
life and greatest efficiency from the machine.

When the machine is run hard day after day around
the clock without any rest—overloaded, overworked
continuously—that's when parts start to break down
and fail. That constant, crushing overload week after
week, month after month, is what causes the machine
to break down completely before it would normally.
That's when the machine *expires* before its time.

The same is true in general for the machine that is
your body. If you're overweight, your machine is overloaded. Your parts (organs) are overworked, over-
burdened, day after day without a letup. If you go on
the Quick Loss Diet and take off 10 to 20 or more
excess pounds in a few weeks, *you're quickly remov-
ing some of the load from your machine, relieving your
heart and other organs.*

You don't burden your heart or the entire machine
by taking away some of the fat load. By lightening the
load, you provide some relief and rest. Even if you
gain back some of the weight after a few weeks, your
machine still had some relief for that lighter-load period. When you diet again and lose weight again, the
machine gets further relief and is better able to function efficiently even if you add weight again later.
With this seesaw pattern, your machine is getting rest
and relief every time the load drops off.

Isn't it just good common sense? The more excess
weight you carry, the harder your heart, other organs,
your entire machine (system) must work to carry that
burden. When you take off some of the fat, your machine has less work to do. It gets some relief, even if
only temporary. This helps the machine until you
eventually get down to your ideal weight or desirable
operating load. Then your machine is able to work

most smoothly and efficiently to achieve its longest operating life.

ARE YOU CHAINED BY FEAR
TO AN IRON BALL?

Consider another parallel to counteract false fears about seesaw reducing or quick losses of weight through dieting. Picture yourself carrying a 20-pound iron ball in your arms for a block. You carry it a second block, a third, a fourth. You either collapse or feel like falling down because the burden is so great and seems so increasingly heavy.

Or—you carry the 20-pound weight for a block. At that point the weight is taken out of your arms and immediately a 10-pound iron ball is substituted. You carry it for the second block. At the start of the third block, the lighter load is replaced by the 20-pound weight. For the fourth block, you change to carrying a 10-pound weight.

What has happened? Obviously you're much fresher and better off with the seesaw exchange of the 10 and 20 pound weights. Every other block, your arms and body and your entire "machine" enjoyed the blessed relief of having your burden cut down by 10 pounds. Your heart didn't have to work harder when it had 10 pounds less to support. On the contrary, it received relief, even though temporary.

By seesawing the weights over the 4 blocks, your machine had to carry and support an average excess weight of 15 pounds instead of a steady burden of 20 pounds. Your body gets the same benefit of carrying a much lower average weight even if it takes you a year to remove that excess fat completely and even if you do it by seesaw reducing.

Certainly it's preferable to take off excess weight swiftly and steadily over a shorter period of time without increases after the initial sharp drop in weight. The primary benefit is that you reach ideal weight faster and thus relieve your "machine" sooner without causing it to accelerate again when weight is added. But I hope you're convinced that if your weight should seesaw because you can't resist going back to overeating after a stringent diet, you need not fear that this will harm your system.

As you'll see in the following chart, even if you lost 20 pounds and then regained it all over a period of four months, you still averaged 10 pounds lower in weight during that period. (The chart is not typical since very few of my patients went right back to their previous excess weight, but here you see what happens even if you did.)

As the chart shows, if this happened to you, that's still 10 pounds less on average that your heart had to drag around for the period. Thus your heart would get some relief and you would feel more health and energy even if only for the limited 4 months time. Of course your goal should be steady loss of weight without sharp upswings.

IF YOU LOST AND THEN REGAINED 20 LBS.
IN FOUR MONTHS...

180   180

AVERAGE WEIGHT 170 LBS. OVER FOUR MONTH PERIOD

160

YOUR HEART HAD 10 FEWER LBS. AVERAGE TO DRAG
AROUND DURING THAT PERIOD

*False Fear: "Won't cutting food intake drastically
hurt me?"*

A fear expressed by many overweights is that
they'll be harmed internally by cutting down food intake severely. I could fill a book with examples showing how wrong this concept is.

Even on semi-starvation and a close to starvation
regimen during wars, few prisoners and others developed heart disease and such impairments from
lack of food. Yet they suffered not only from starvation
portions of poor quality foods, they also had to endure
miserable living conditions, lack of sanitation, severe
beatings, relentless interrogation, physical and mental
tortures and worse.

The eating of the general populations in most European countries dropped drastically during World War
II. Many people lacked proteins, vitamins, meats and
fats. Instead of growing weak and sick, most adults became healthier. They often lost their hypertension,
shortness of breath, gallbladder disease, and many
other debilitating disorders.

Hospital statistics in many countries—Holland and
Norway for example—showed a 40% decrease in
heart disease during the war, along with the sharp
drop in food consumption and resultant general weight
reduction. After the war ended and food became
more plentiful, many people went back to their old
habits of overeating and thus piling on excess fat. The
percentages of those with heart disease and the other
ills mentioned rose along with the increase in food
consumption. By 1949 the tables on high incidence of
coronary diseases and serious physical disorders were
right back up where they had been in 1941.

Instead of worrying about being harmed by cutting
down sharply on your food intake with a quick reducing diet, you'd better concentrate on the serious harm
you're doing yourself if you're eating too much and

carrying around that awful, debilitating burden of excess weight.

A doctor placed eleven obese patients on a fasting diet of nothing but water, vitamins and minerals—no food at all. They fasted from *12 to 117 days*. None of them could "sneak in" any food as they were under constant watch in the hospital. All of them were in far better physical condition when reduced than when the fasting diets started.

That supervised fasting (definitely not recommended except under doctor's orders) was to help the very heavy person get down to normal or near normal as quickly as possible and then proceed to Stay Slim Eating.

False Fear: "Won't unbalanced dieting and changing my eating habits hurt me?"

Many people fear that changing their eating habits or going on an "unbalanced" diet will be harmful. They ignore the fact that their so-called "balanced" eating habits produced the excess weight which ruins good looks and impairs health. Many have told me, "I'm afraid that I'll be weak, dizzy, that I'll have 'hunger headaches' and worse."

When you are on any special diet, if you experience such undesirable symptoms and they don't disappear in a few days, your doctor should check your condition. In my experience, most of the people who complain of "hunger headaches" and other such symptoms are the ones who have lost the least weight or none at all. In other words, they're experiencing ill effects even before the diet has really started or while cheating on the diet.

A popular story tells of a man complaining bitterly to a friend about his new diet. His friend asked, "How long have you been on the diet?" The man answered, "I start tomorrow." This is not untypical of the complaining dieter.

The great majority of my patients who lose up to 10 pounds on the Quick Loss Diet the first week, and 3 to 7 pounds a week thereafter, usually comment "No bad symptoms at all. No weakness. No headaches. Never felt better in my life."

I've found that only a tiny percentage, from 1 to 3 of every 100 patients on quick reducing diets actually feel undesirable symptoms, a much lower percentage than on "balanced" diets. Whether real or imagined, such reactions must be treated with understanding. Usually the "symptoms" disappear after another day or two on the diet.

However, if an individual is mentally disturbed and his serenity and sanity are at stake with dieting, then obesity is to be preferred. This is not true of the overwhelming majority of overweights. For them a change in eating habits and an "unbalanced," restricted diet is most healthful, not harmful.

Some people insist, like one patient: "I'm naturally heavy and it's bad for me to be slim." This is sheer self-deceit, unworthy of the intelligent person. In all my years of medical practice, I've never examined a normal person whom I've found to be healthier for being overweight than at ideal or average weight.

Another woman protested, "Losing a lot of weight lowers my resistance and causes a lot more colds and other illnesses." Patient after patient has used this as an excuse for staying fat. I keep emphasizing that getting excess fat off the stomach, pancreas, liver, heart and other organs is most *helpful*. The entire system functions better. Colds and other ills are reduced rather than increased.

My experience with thousands of patients proves to me conclusively that colds and other sickness are reduced as you reduce your weight. Your own good sense, plus the factual evidence, should prove to you that this is so. Does a truck motor run better when overloaded? Of course not. It wheezes and groans, parts break and finally the engine stops functioning. The same is true of the human overloaded with fat.

Another fallacy is the common statement, "It's better to have a little extra fat on the body as a reserve for illness." Actually every pound of overweight burdens the human system and impairs its functioning. The organs have the extra drag of feeding and carrying that "extra layer" of fat. This impairs rather than helps the body in fighting illness.

If you elect to overeat and stay fat in spite of the hazards, that's up to you. Just don't delude yourself that you're healthier when fat. If you should ever decide to take off the extra blubber and get down to your ideal weight, your wonderful new sense of well-being and extra lightness and vigor will be your best proof that you're healthier when slim.

False Fear: "Won't dieting bring on vitamin deficiency?"

This fear of dangerous vitamin deficiency is a common excuse for people afraid of dieting in general and quick-loss dieting in particular. Even though millions in this country are deprived of enough food or the proper foods, there is very little evidence of actual vitamin deficiency.

Dr. William Daniel Herbert, associate in medicine at the Harvard Medical School, stated, "When all the cases of vitamin deficiency reported in the United States in a single year are added up, they do not reach the figure of 20,000, and therefore the clinically ascertainable incidence, as manifested by published reports, is much less than one percent of the U.S. population: 20,000 projected into a figure of 180,000,000." (Actually one-tenth of one percent.)

There is no real chance of developing vitamin deficiency on the Quick Loss or other diets in this book. Don't be fooled by propagandists who imply that peo-

ple can be "vitamin-starved" even on 3 meals a day.
Such vitamin deficiency is theoretical only. In spite
of that, I suggest that while dieting you take any common once-daily vitamin and mineral product. On a
fasting type of diet of only 300 to 400 calories daily,
take a stronger "therapeutic" vitamin product.

False Fear: "Won't I look scrawny, haggard and
   out of proportion if I lose weight quickly?"

Another common excuse for not taking off weight is
the expressed fear, "Even if I'm fat, I look strong and
healthy now. I'm afraid to diet because I'll look weak
and sickly. My skin will sag. The weight will come off
in the wrong places and I'll look all out of proportion."

This is an outright fake excuse. Down deep most of
those who use it are aware of its falsity. All of us
know too many overweight men and women who
looked "the picture of health" and suddenly took sick
or died. It has been proved thoroughly by statistics
that looking meaty and even "pleasingly plump" is
not a healthy look.

When you lose weight rapidly, your skin soon firms
to normal proportions. About the only thing that sags
on you are your oversized clothes. When people slim
down they're invariably complimented on the radiant
new look of fitness and beauty. It's an old-fashioned,
outmoded idea that you should have "meat on your
bones." The shocking facts about illness and earlier
death among overweights, stated later, should dispel
any lingering notion that a heavy look is a healthy
look.

As for fat "coming off in the wrong places," this is
another fallacy. Overweight is overweight wherever
it is located on your body. When you reduce, the
weight comes off all over in time. If much of your
weight is in your chest or neck, abdomen, pelvis,
thighs or calves, you must nevertheless keep going
for total reduction of weight. The loss of weight may

be greatest in areas where you're less concerned about losing it, but eventually weight loss is proportionate to your natural conformations.

If you reduce and keep your weight down, you'll eventually be rewarded by losing weight where you wish, as much as is possible. If your legs, for example, are naturally heavy, loss of weight will reduce them to a minimum but you can't expect them ever to be really thin. At ideal weight, you'll have your most pleasing proportions possible.

False Fear: "I'm afraid I won't succeed."

I can promise you from my experience with thousands of different types of overweights that many who have failed before succeed with Quick Loss dieting as recommended here. As I've shown, even if you lose weight and gain some of it back, your body, heart and other organs get the relief of comparative rest at least during the period when you were slimmer. You have everything to gain except pounds by trying my recommendations. Every minute of doubt you may have is a minute wasted.

To summarize, the big plus working for you to succeed with the Quick Weight Loss method, even if you've failed in dieting before, is the sharp loss of weight the first week. It proves quickly that you can succeed. Also helping you is the fact that your appetite decreases as the fat comes off. You break the habit of overeating. The overwhelming desire for rich food is usually gone. Your eating habits have changed for the better.

10. ADDITIONAL REDUCING QUICK TIPS AND SPECIAL AIDS

Over the years I've found that a number of simple "quick-tips" have helped former overweights to keep from letting excess fat creep up on them again. Some of these aids are noted elsewhere in this book, but bear brief repetition as helpful reminders and additional methods for staying slim.

More Activity, Less Sleep. You have a better chance to become slim and stay at ideal weight if you limit your sleeping to a maximum of 8 hours out of every 24. There are several reasons. Activity, alertness, keeping on the go, all make reducing easier, as you use more energy and calories. You're less likely to eat unnecessarily because of listlessness and boredom.

When you're sleeping, you don't assist your body as much in burning up the food you've eaten. You usually use up to 3 times as many calories when awake and on the move than when asleep, as shown by the following averaged figures. While not universally accurate, these figures are helpful as a guide to general minimal utilization of calories.

MEN:

8 hours work, mostly standing ..	1200 cals.
1 hour activity getting ready for work	180
6 hours activity after work, walking, sitting, etc.	720

1 hour activity preparatory to re-
tiring 180

8 hours bed rest (sleep) (aver-
age) 540

Total calories used 2820

WOMEN:

8 hours household activities 880

8 hours walking, sitting, resting 720

8 hours bed rest (sleep) 480

Total calories used 2080

Note that many more calories per hour are burned
up when awake and active than when asleep or resting
abed. In effect, you deposit calories in your personal
bank with the food you eat. You withdraw the calories
by using up energy at work and play. If you deposit
more calories than you withdraw, the fat deposits increase and your weight goes up. It's as simple as that.

The longer you sleep beyond 8 hours daily, the more
likely that you'll put on excess weight as you fail to
use up calories from the food you've eaten during the
day. The more active you are—working, walking,
swimming, bicycling, bowling, golfing and other pursuits—the more food calories you use up and the fewer
will be left to settle in fat depots in your body.

Of course if you eat more and take in 200 calories
of food for each 100 calories of energy expenditure,
you'll keep your excess weight and increase it no matter how active you are. Even if you use up 3,500 calories daily, if you take in 4,500 calories of food you're
depositing 1,000 excess calories that day to add fat
to your body.

Eat Slowly and you'll be satisfied with less food. Cut
your food into many small portions, then take small
mouthfuls and chew slowly and thoroughly before
swallowing. Don't gulp liquids either, drink them

slowly, s-t-r-e-t-c-h out a glass of skim milk or any other beverage or food—it will seem like more. Don't be a food bolter.

If you're having a banana and cottage cheese for lunch, for example, don't just peel the banana and eat it whole. Instead, cut the banana into many small slices and ring them around the cottage cheese on lettuce leaves. Eating slowly, you now have the feeling of eating a more substantial meal. Do the same with any fruit, even as an interval snack.

Don't Eat or Reach for Food Unless You're Hungry. Remember how many times you've been disgusted with yourself when you've eaten something you didn't have to, didn't really want to. A neighbor stops in and you have a muffin (140 c.) with your coffee that you hadn't intended to eat. Or at the office you stop just for coffee and find that you've swallowed a doughnut (135 c.) without being at all hungry.

Before you reach for any food ask yourself whether you're really hungry. *If not, don't eat it.* Eating only when hungry can result in the elimination of many hundreds of calories daily. At meals, cease eating as soon as your hunger stops, don't keep eating just for the sake of eating or to finish the food on your plate.

Less Food on Your Plate. It has been my personal observation, and the experience of patients, that if you put less food on your plate, you're less tempted to eat more than is necessary to soothe your hunger. The reverse is also true. If you put more cottage cheese or meat or other food on your plate than you really could do with, you're likely to finish the excess anyhow. It may amount to only one more meatball or just a tablespoon more of cottage cheese or an extra slice of bread, but it all adds up to extra calories you didn't need and wouldn't have consumed otherwise. It's practically a rule—the less on the plate, the less is eaten.

Before Each Meal when you're dieting, drink a glass or cup or more of water, tea, coffee or non-caloric beverages. Just this little trick of pouring in the liquid *first,* is amazingly helpful in giving you a sense of fullness and in decreasing hunger pangs so that you're satisfied to eat less. You may finish the meal with a non-caloric beverage, and drink during the meal also. Every swallow helps fill you up without adding calories.

Omit Salt or use it sparingly. Salted foods tend to retain more water in the body and increase weight. Unsalted foods are less tempting and you eat less.

Don't Use Sugar in Beverages. Every teaspoonful adds 18 calories. If you ordinarily use 2 teaspoonfuls of sugar in coffee, for instance, and drink 4 cupfuls a day, you're adding 144 calories of sugar alone. Non-caloric sugar substitutes now are just as sweetening. You get plenty of carbohydrates and energy from the other foods you usually eat during the day.

Use Salads Abundantly when permitted on your particular diet (not permitted on the Quick Weight Loss Diet, for example). Ten large leaves of lettuce are only 25 calories. Using them as a tossed salad with non-caloric dressing makes a very filling and satisfying food as a snack or part of a meal.

Never Use Butter, margarine, oil, cream, fats, mayonnaise and rich dressings unless prescribed on your diet. If you use 2 pats of butter at each meal (as too many overweights do), that totals 300 calories a day. Two tablespoons of mayonnaise on a salad adds 220 calories. Two tablespoons of cream in a cup of coffee, 4 cups a day, adds 280 calories (with 2 teaspoons of sugar per cup that totals 424 calories with coffee which alone has no calories at all).

Small Calorie Savings Save Pounds. You can lose
5–10–15–20 pounds in one year by eating the same
foods as usual but cutting down on 2 or 3 items which
you certainly won't miss. If you cut 50 calories a day,
you save 18,250 calories in a year. There are about
3,500 calories to each pound, amounting to a saving
of 5.2 pounds in a year.

To cut out 50 calories daily, eliminate 3 teaspoons
of sugar (use non-caloric sweetening instead), or ¾
slice of bread, or 1 level teaspoon of butter. Thus you
save 5.2 pounds a year very easily.

You can take 100 calories off your daily intake by
cutting out 1 slice of bread and 2 teaspoons of sugar,
or 1 straight alcoholic drink, or 1 glass of whole milk,
or 1 glass of beer, or 1 glass of sugary soda (drink non-
caloric instead). This slight change means 10.4 pounds
less in the year.

Want to try for 150 calories saved per day? Eliminate 1 slice of bread and butter, or 1 martini or high-
ball, or 1 tablespoon of rich salad dressing (use low-
calorie dressing instead). Now you've saved 15.6
pounds during the year by this cutdown alone.

For those who put on weight slowly, hardly realizing it, this cutdown system is a simple form of natural
reducing help in your Stay Slim Eating. However you
must not replace the eliminated items with other indulgences.

If you now do a little more walking, golfing, bicycling or other such exercise daily, you may save another 5 pounds over the year.

Avoid Concentrated Rich Foods. Watch out for
those high-calorie concentrated foods in the listing
and skip them. If you pass up 4 tablespoons of hollandaise sauce on asparagus, for instance, you eliminate
200 calories (6 stalks of asparagus without butter or
any sauce are only about 25 calories). Look down the
calorie list and familiarize yourself with high-calorie
concentrated foods to avoid, such as pork sausage (4

oz.—340 c.), baked beans (1 cup—320), candied sweet potatoes (medium—295), dates (pitted, 1 cup—505), chocolate layer cake (2″ sector—420), peanuts (shelled, ½ cup—420) and others. Surely it isn't worth using up 20% or so of your day's caloric allowance with a handful of peanuts or another unnecessary high-calorie food.

Taste the Forbidden Food but don't eat it. There's no need to deny yourself a taste of something you find particularly delicious, but remember that a taste has only a fraction of the calories of a portion. For instance at a party you might sample 1 small hors d'oeuvre to compliment your hostess, but if you eat one after another every time the trays are passed, you can easily consume over 1,000 calories *even before dinner starts.*

Break Up Your Meal, save some for later. Remember the previous advice to stop eating when your hunger stops. Put aside whatever you haven't eaten for a snack later or for the next day. Many of my patients tell me that this one tip has saved them hundreds of calories daily.

Speak Up: "I'm Dieting." Don't hesitate to tell your hostess or people you're lunching or dining with that you're on a diet and must skip certain foods and have small portions of others. You can admire a dessert and compliment your hostess on how delicious it looks, but tell her firmly, "I'm on a diet for my health and I can't afford to cheat. I must pass up the beautiful dessert."

You can explain the same way to business associates at lunch when you skip a cocktail. Chances are they'll admire your fortitude and wish they could emulate it.

It's not much of a hostess or host who feels "insulted" because you pass up calorie-rich offerings or take

smaller portions. After all, something very important
is at stake—*your health and longer life*. It's far better
to speak up than to be weighed down by dangerous
fat.

Use Low-Calorie Substitutes. One of your greatest
aids to reducing and staying slim is to use the excellent low-calorie food substitutes that are fairly new
and improving all the time. More and more packages
are available to you with the calories marked, like a
combination of tomato soup, beef stew and peaches,
"a full 3-course meal, less than 300 calories."

Tasty salad dressings are available with practically
no calories, instead of over 100 calories per tablespoon. A sugar-free gelatin dessert has only 10 calories
a serving, compared with 200 calories per serving of
ice cream. There are many more such calorie-saving
opportunities.

With all the fine sugar substitutes there's no reason
to use sugar at 18 calories per teaspoon, about 770
calories per cup.

Non-caloric carbonated beverages are a great aid.
You can drink bottle after bottle, be refreshed and
absorb hardly a calorie. Save about 100 calories per
8 oz. glass compared with sugary soda.

When Eating in Restaurants: Today you can eat out
in most any restaurant and still keep your calorie intake low. Keep in mind the tips and calorie tables
in this book and use your good judgment, pause and
choose, don't just order the first thing on the menu or
that comes to your mind.

For example, in Stay Slim Eating, skip rich ap-
petizers and creamed soups. Instead you can start
with shrimps with a little cocktail sauce, or clear soup,
clam broth (not clam chowder) or consomme. For
your main course, choose meat, poultry or fish, not
fried. Have it brought without gravy or butter sauce,
no butter on any of the food, no creamed vegetables.

If you have a salad, have them leave off rich dressing; instead add a little vinegar or fresh lime or lemon juice. No bread or rolls.

Skip the dessert or have at most a half grapefruit, other fresh fruit or gelatin dessert. Have plenty of tea or coffee during and after the meal, without milk, cream or sugar.

Choosing in this fashion is easy enough and you won't seem like a freak. When you stop feeling hungry, stop eating; have the leftover food taken away. An increasing number of restaurants have low-calorie specials. For instance, one of the finest hotels in New York had on the menu as their low-calorie special: Lean leg of lamb, asparagus without hollandaise, lettuce and sliced tomato without dressing—under 200 calories. They also offered leg of lamb with creamed cauliflower, baked potato with butter and sour cream sauce, salad and roquefort dressing, and rolls and butter—over 600 calories.

Whenever it's not impolite, don't linger at the table. Get up, go into another room or take a walk. Of course you're less likely to eat when there's no food in front of you.

If you have lunch at the same restaurant daily, you can have them keep low-calorie foods for your convenience. Above all, take special care with everything you order. Even if it's only a hamburger, tell them to broil it without butter or fats, and not to give you a butter-soaked bun. These seemingly small caloric savings can save you extra pounds each week.

No Second Helpings. The second helping is one of the greatest curses in eating at home or as a guest, and you must make it one of your strictest rules to avoid this. Tell your wife or mother or hostess courteously but firmly, "No thanks, no second helpings, I'm on a strict diet, please help me keep it."

I have been appalled, after hearing a wife say virtuously to her husband, "Nothing for you for dinner

but lean roast beef and sliced tomatoes," to see her
then pile on another slice of roast beef and another as
soon as the man's plate was clean. Then she tells
friends, "I can't understand why Henry keeps gaining
weight, I feed him only lean meats, vegetables and
salads." Those second (and third and fourth) helpings
will wreck most any diet.

Limit System. Limit yourself ahead of time by what
you put on your plate, particularly when you're having
a snack. If you're having cookies and non-caloric soda,
put 1 or 2 small cookies on your plate, *then put the
rest away*. Out of sight is out of stomach. Invariably
if you leave the cookies or cheese or other tasty foods
in front of you, there's a good chance you'll keep
gobbling mouthfuls—often without even realizing that
you're eating.

Chewing Gum Helps Some. I find that many of my
patients have skipped their usual calorie-filled snacks
by chewing on gum instead. It may help you, and you
can even get artificially sweetened gum, although there
are few enough calories in an ordinary stick. You
might also try dietetic gumdrops made with sugar
substitute.

Hard Candy Snack? Some people are able to as-
suage a craving by having a small piece of hard candy.
That's fine if you stop with one small piece once or
twice a day. But what may happen is that you don't
stop with one piece. A friend told me about three overweight secretaries in his office who had read that a
piece of hard candy will kill hunger pangs. They kept
a dish filled with hard candy on a table in the office.
Each night the dish was empty and the girls were
fuller and fatter. Instead of substituting one hard
candy for other foods, they were *adding* a load of sugar
calories to their regular calorie-rich meals.

Keep a Calorie and Weight Diary. It's been a great help to many of my patients to carry a little pad or slip of paper and keep track of the number of calories they consume meal by meal. When you write it down on paper that way you're more likely to stay within your daily limit and stop eating when you've reached it.

Also write down what you weighed each morning upon arising. You're much encouraged on the Quick Loss Diet to see your weight in writing diminish rapidly each day. On the other hand, when you're on Stay Slim Eating, if your weight is going up day by day as you record it, you see "the handwriting on the wall" and you cut down or go on the Quick Loss Diet again.

Zero-Calorie Items. Keep in mind these items which contain zero or few calories and can be used as often as you wish on most diets (where not contraindicated):

Carbonated beverages, non-caloric
Clear soups, consomme, bouillon
Herbs and spices, horseradish
Lemon and lime juice
Seltzer, club soda
Tea and coffee
Vinegar
Spices

Use Low-Calorie Vegetables. These are excellent foods which you may use in quantity unless not permitted (as on the Quick Loss Diet). Don't use butter or fats on the vegetables or in their preparation. The lowest-calorie vegetables are in the 5% list, a little higher calories in the 10% list, and the highest—but still relatively low-calorie foods—in the 15%–20% listing.

5%:

Asparagus	Celery	Lettuce	Sauerkraut
Bean sprouts	Chard	Mushrooms	Spinach
Beet greens	Cucumbers	Parsley	Squash, summer
Broccoli	Endive	Pimentos	String beans
Cabbage	Escarole	Peppers (green, red)	Watercress
Cauliflower	Kale	Radishes	

10%:

Bamboo shoots	Carrots	Leeks	Tomatoes
Beets	Eggplant	Okra	Turnips
Brussels sprouts	Kohlrabi	Scallions	

15–20%:

Artichokes	Parsnips	Pumpkin
Onions	Peas	Squash, winter

Selective Dairy Products. Skim milk, cottage cheese, pot cheese, farmer cheese and cultured buttermilk should be kept in mind as excellent reducing aids and helps in staying slim (unless not permitted on your diet). These foods are relatively low in calories, considering their nutritive elements. Every time you drink a glass of skim milk (90) instead of whole milk (165) you save 75 calories, the difference being primarily in fats.

At first you may miss the richer flavor, but then you will probably prefer skim to the "rich and fatty" taste of whole milk when sampled again. (An interesting sidelight is provided by a noted animal breeder who states that the most prized veal at the finest restaurants is from his skim-milk-fed calves.)

Diet a Meal at a Time. One trick used by some of my dieters is to keep the calories down for one meal at a time and not worry about the rest. For instance, you concentrate on your low-calorie breakfast, not giving any thought to being deprived of rich foods at lunch. Then you stick to a low-calorie lunch, not worrying about breaking down at dinner. At dinner, you maintain your restricted diet and you're through the day. But if you asked yourself on awakening, "How am I ever going to abstain through 3 meals, or through a whole day?" you might have broken your resolution at breakfast.

The alcoholic is advised similarly by Alcoholics Anonymous not to worry that he'll never be able to drink again all his life, but instead to concentrate on the resolution, "I will not have a drink *today.*"

Picture Yourself. When an overweight patient first comes to me I urge that she have a snapshot taken of herself (or himself), preferably in a bathing suit. Then as she reduces she can compare her figure in the mirror every few days with the one in the photo. With the Quick Loss Diet, the difference is often excitingly apparent after only a week. Carry a "before" snapshot and let your vanity take over to keep you from going back to being the horrible example in the picture.

It has been said that more diets have begun on bathing beaches and in dress shops than in doctors' offices. Some overweights have also helped themselves while reducing by buying a dress or suit that's too tight. Then they find that they work harder to take off the pounds and inches in order to fit into the new clothing properly and attractively.

Reward Yourself. You may find it helpful to follow

the "reward system" used successfully by some of my patients. One young woman said that every time she was tempted to stop at a soda fountain or coffee shop for a snack, she'd conquer the temptation and put the money she would have spent into a "reward envelope" in her purse. When the change turned into dollars she'd buy herself a new article of clothing that she felt otherwise would be an extravagance but which she wanted very much. Saving those dollars and spending them made good sense in respect to her improved health and appearance as she slimmed down.

A family in my care with four members who were all overweight went on a "charity diet." For a month they put aside all the money they'd saved on costly desserts, liquors and other expensive and fatty foods. They then gave the kitty to their favorite charity. They continued on this charity diet because they found it rewarding to the spirit as well as to the figure.

Instead-Of's. When you "must" have a snack in your Stay Slim Eating, keep in mind this list of possible snack foods that are relatively low in calories and can be taken *instead of* the high-calorie food you'd reach for without thinking.

Apple—70
Buttermilk—90
Cantaloupe, half—40
Carrot, raw—20
Cottage, pot, farmer
 cheese, 1 oz.—30
Cucumber—25
Gelatin, sugar-free—10

Grapefruit, half—55
Orange—65
Plum—30
Radishes (4),—12
Shrimps (4),—40
Tomato juice—50
Coffee, tea, non-caloric
 soda—0

Compare this with drinking sugar-rich sodas and whole milk; eating cake, cookies, ice cream, nuts, pie, pudding. You'll save hundreds of calories per snack by substituting the "instead-of"—for example, a half grapefruit, 55, instead of chocolate layer cake, 365 calories—saving 310 calories in one snack.

Don't Feed a Cold. There's no advantage really in the old adage, "Feed a cold and starve a fever." If you stuff yourself with food, whether you have a cold or a fever or not, you're putting an extra burden on your organs rather than helping them. If you have a fever, there's no disadvantage in eating normally. It all depends on your hunger. Most often the appetite diminishes with a cold or fever or both. You have nothing to gain except discomfort if you force food when not hungry.

Start Quick Loss Dieting at Once. If you're overweight, realize that there's no "special time" for starting. The best time is now. If you delay, you're already beginning to lose the battle. No diet can reduce you while you think about it, you must go on it. The sooner you start, the quicker you'll lose weight, the better you'll feel and look. Have no fear of withdrawal symptoms such as experienced by those who go off cigarettes, alcohol and drugs. With Quick Loss dieting the only thing you lose is the excessive craving for food, soon after you start.

Cheating Test. On the Quick Loss Diet (also on high-fat and fasting diets), a simple test will show whether or not you're following instructions as you should. Get a powder called acetest at a drug store. When a drop of urine is placed on the powder it will turn purple if you're dieting correctly. But if you're cheating, the drop on the powder will remain white. This test has helped some of my patients turn honest with their dieting and lose weight more quickly and steadily.

Carry Your Quick Loss Diet and Calorie Chart. Keep an extra copy of the Quick Weight Loss Diet and

the Calorie Count Listing with you. If you're on one
of the other diets, copy it on a sheet of paper to carry.
Referring to the instructions every time you eat will
help you diet exactly as you should and lose weight
most quickly.

A Dieting Buddy Helps. Children who are learning
to swim at camp are helped by having a "water buddy"
who is learning at the same time and the same stage.
You may find it helpful, as others have, to diet along
with an overweight friend. You can compare weight
losses and check on each other to stay in line.

I know of twin brothers who were both about 30
pounds overweight. They went on diets the same day.
At the end of each week, one twin would have to
give the other a dollar for every pound he weighed
more than his brother. When they were both at desired
weight months later, each had won in better health
and appearance.

Weigh Yourself Daily. As urged before, get on the
bathroom scale each morning upon arising. If you see
that 3-pound danger signal, go back on the Quick Loss
Diet without delay.

Use Seasonings to Spice Up Diets. A man complained to a friend, "My wife is a confirmed weight-
watcher. My problem is that the weight she's watching
is *mine!*" If you're the cook of the family, one way
you can help silence such complaints is to spice up
low-calorie servings so that their flavor brings a smile
instead of a frown. If you "try a little harder," you'll
find that it isn't too difficult to improve low-calorie
foods from a taste viewpoint.

For instance, here are some suggestions from a very
fine cook:

Boiled carrots, which are very low in calories, become much more delicious when you sprinkle them
with grated or chopped, fresh mint leaves.

Use of monosodium glutamate products, now available in containers like salt, helps perk up the flavors of low-calorie vegetables, lean meats and fish.

Chopped parsley and chives add a very tasty touch to plain boiled potatoes and other vegetables. This fresh flavor is easy to achieve now since parsley and chives are sold in small freezer packages. Also you can grow them on any sunny windowsill. Clip and use the top inch and the plants grow right back again for further use and enjoyment.

Oregano and other flavorful Italian seasonings and spices sparkle up plain green beans and other good low-calorie vegetables.

Instead of using regular salt, which is better left out of most diets, make low-calorie foods more satisfying with no-sodium salt substitutes. You can get them most anywhere now. Also, don't overlook the use of "seasoned salt" made without sodium.

Juicy, fresh lemon wedges on the plate or table, a pretty little flagon of herb vinegar, other no-calorie aids, all help keep the dieter *on* the diet instead of slipping off.

There are dozens, even hundreds, of excellent, tasty relishes which improve low-calorie meals from a flavor viewpoint. These can be used in moderation at most any meal without adding too many calories. Of course, good sense and judgment must be your guide. If you eat sweet pickle or many other relishes by the heaping tablespoonful (as I've seen some gluttons do), the calories will pile up. You'll be cheating yourself.

If a quick weight loss diet allows you the use of relish, that means a little relish for flavoring, not a full-sized portion like another vegetable. If you over-indulge in relishes meal after meal, don't say, "That diet doesn't work." Instead, blame yourself for not working at your diet fairly and intelligently.

The same caution goes for all the flavoring tips in this book. Their purpose is to help the dieter enjoy his restricted portions thoroughly. If the result is to *in-*

crease the portions or lead the dieter to grab second helpings, then it's better for his reducing success and good health to leave the foods bland and relatively flavorless. Nothing must be permitted to block the way to that one primary goal—*to get that weight off.*

Keep a Refrigerator Diet-Snack Container Full. A lovely woman patient told me that she finally came to me determined to take off her excess 35 pounds when her husband kept calling her "a *barrel* of fun." She went on, "I had been thinking that my friends regarded me as a happy-go-lucky companion. When my eyes were opened I realized that they considered me a fat clown."

She stayed with the Quick Weight Loss Diet so faithfully that within a couple of months she slimmed down to become the most attractive wife in her social set. She told me that now, on her stay-slim eating, she finds that this is a help:

She took a short, pretty glass vase and painted on it "Stay Slim Snacks." She keeps this in her refrigerator filled with water (changed frequently) and a variety of carrot and celery sticks. Similarly, in small glass jars labeled the same way, she has handy low-calorie nibbles such as radishes and fresh, spiced (no oil) mushrooms.

All these snacks contain practically no calories. When she finds herself about to reach for a cookie or candy or other high-calorie snack, she heads for the refrigerator instead. Now her healthful impulse is to reach for a carrot stick instead of a chocolate-covered cherry. She emphasizes that the important point is to keep those "stay slim snacks" containers filled so that they're always at fingertip reach for instant snacking.

Guard Against Food and Diet "Myths" That Lead You Astray. Many people have the craziest notions about what constitutes "healthful eating." Often the food myths have been fostered by constant, costly propaganda by special interests or misguided "food and nutrition experts." A patient and her overweight teenage daughter invariably failed in dieting because the mother believed firmly that everyone in the family had to start the day with a "big, hot breakfast." That's utter nonsense.

For the overweight, a breakfast of a chilled half-cantaloupe and artificially sweetened coffee or tea is far more healthful than the traditional bowl of steaming cereal bathed in hot butter, heaped wih sugar or doused with whole milk or cream. It's infinitely better for you than a stack of calorie-rich pancakes, or a platter of ham and eggs swimming in butter with a side dish of greasy homefries.

Even for the overweight youngster, a small ball of ice cream and nothing else would be a more healthful breakfast since it would total fewer calories than those traditional "heaping hot breakfast" specialties. As for nutrition, there's as much or more desirable food value and energy in a bowl of high-protein cold cereal with skim milk, as in a similar serving of a hot cereal with butter and whole milk or cream.

It's all a matter of your own good sense as a guide. If you enjoy hot cereal, have it with skim milk or plain with artificial sweetening. That's better for you than if you add the high butter and cream calories.

Another common myth is that artificially sweetened canned fruits and other foods are less nutritious than the same varieties in heavy sugar syrup. This simply is not true. You get enough "energy" from other natural foods so that you don't need the sugar calories. By eating the artificially sweetened foods you lose only a load of fat-producing calories, not any vital nutritional elements. Once down to your ideal weight, your stay-slim eating can include sugar if you desire it, as long as you stay within the prescribed daily calorie intake.

If you continue to believe in the aforementioned and the many other misconceptions which lead you to add calories for the sake of nutrition, you're willfully deluding yourself and harming your health and appearance. That goes for the whole family. If you're in doubt at any time, look up the scientific facts about a food, instead of being misled blindly by false clichés or advice of health faddists who frequently have some angle for personal gain.

Another misconception is that *steam baths* are a marvelous quick aid in reducing. This is false. A fat man may contend that he has stepped on a scale before and after a steam bath and seen an actual drop of several pounds. The explanation is that such loss is due to an outpouring of water, not fat. The water has been released in the process of perspiring heavily.

This weight loss is strictly temporary. The pounds go right back on in a few hours, as the scales would show if the same kind of comparison was made later. If you find a steam bath relaxing, if it makes you "feel good," then enjoy it. But don't count on it as a dependable reducing aid. The same goes for body massage. There's no other way: You must change your eating habits meaningfully in order to enjoy quick and *continuing* weight loss.

Perhaps the most prevalent and disheartening myth of all, I must stress again and again, is the terrible misconception that the only "right way to reduce" is by losing one or two pounds a week, and that it's dangerous to lose a pound or more a day. I have before me a typical article from a national magazine read by more than 10 million people monthly. It gives a "sensible, balanced diet" and concludes that this "brings a safe and satisfying loss of about 1½ pounds a week."

So far as I'm concerned, based on over 40 years of actual experience in reducing overweights, such statements are utterly *fraudulent* . . . even though not intentionally so. The misguided overweight, especially the very heavy individual, will fail miserably on such a diet when he sees that he only loses one or two pounds a week.

He is being cheated when he is told that such a method will work for him. Yet, too many so-called nutritional experts, and even physicians without much experience of reducing patients in their practices, adhere obstinately and blindly to that outmoded viewpoint. Meanwhile those overweights fail again and again to reduce, and they moan, "I'm one of those unfortunates who just can't get the fat off."

You can see for yourself in one short week that there's no "myth" about the Quick Weight Loss Diet. It will do the one, all-important thing that the "sensible, balanced" diets fail to do—*it will get that weight off*. It will do this with the encouraging speed that is absolutely essential to reducing success for the vast majority of overweights. It will conclusively explode the other myth that you're one of those "unfortunates" who can't get the fat off.

Realize what a different quick weight loss makes from the standpoint of the dieter's morale, your own mental outlook: If you're an overweight man tipping the scale at 190 pounds, you'll lose 9 to 19 pounds the first week, if you're faithful to this diet which permits you a restricted variety of fine foods. If you're a heavy woman weighing 150 pounds, you'll lose 7 to 15 pounds the first week on this safe, pleasant method of eating.

The sooner you rid your mind of the misconception that slow reducing is the only safe reducing, the quicker you'll take off the pounds. In no time at all you'll start seeing real encouragement in the mirror, as well as practically overnight on the scale. You'll be delighted to note the visible, sure signs that you'll soon reach the slim, attractive, youthful body buried under all the layers of unhealthy, burdensome fat.

Join a Reducing Club? Yes and No. Reducing clubs banding together a number of men or women, or both, with the common goal of losing weight, keep springing up in various communities. Such a club can accomplish lasting good in helping you to reduce if the members are guided by the right reducing methods. I've encouraged groups of individuals to diet together as a "club" with regular meetings.

It's a real help when compatible people can get together weekly and compare the weight losses which are such heartening and *necessary* phases in arriving at the goal. As the members weigh in and are measured, they're ashamed if they haven't lost since the previous meeting. A lady gets a thrill of pride if the numbers show that she has done better than others.

An excellent system is to form a Quick Weight Loss Club which goes on the Quick Weight Loss Diet for the first few weeks. Then the members vote to switch together to the all-fruit diet for a week, back on the QWL Diet, then a week on the all-vegetable diet, back on QWL for a week, and so on. It's fun to arrive at a consensus of which quick reducing diet most members want each week after the first few on QWL. Later meetings help the individuals to maintain their ideal weight on Stay Slim Eating, with an occasional return to a week on the Quick Weight Loss Diet.

You must realize, as some overweights do not, that just joining a "reducing club" is no guarantee that you'll lose pounds. If a club is based on "slow, balanced dieting" principles, as too many are, plus a little group calisthenics, the rewards may be social, but that's all.

A discouraged husband, deeply upset about his formerly attractive wife's gross overweight, told me, "She thought she'd solved everything by joining a reducing club for dieting and exercise. They ate more at the meetings or at the kaffee-klatch afterwards, than they would if they'd stayed at home. All they really exercised were their mouths."

He went on unhappily, "They keep kidding themselves. My wife said that at the last meeting one

member reported, 'Yes, I lost weight last week. I went
down from 150 to 149 9/10.'"

Hopeless, after belonging to the misguided reducing
club for two months, this same woman visited me at
her husband's insistence. She lost 10 pounds her first
week on the Quick Weight Loss Diet. She was excited
and encouraged. She was on her way to saving her
marriage. She could have done the same in the reducing club with the same effective method, but never on
slow and unsure dieting.

Don't Worry About Food Content, Only Calories.
I learned in her first visit that a patient, who had never
succeeded previously in dieting, was blocked primarily
by an overabundance of empty knowledge about foods
and nutrition. She considered herself an expert and
immediately let me know it. She said, "I know all
about proper dieting so I don't think you can really
help me. I understand full well that I must keep the
carbohydrates down, the proteins up, the cholesterol
down but the calcium up, the—"

I interrupted, "The only important thing you have
to know eventually is the calorie content of foods.
You don't have to even know that until you go on
Stay Slim Eating later. I'm going to start you on my
Stillman Quick Weight Loss Diet where you don't even
count calories, you just follow the simple, clear guides."

It's too true that "a little knowledge can be dangerous" in dieting. Another patient said, "I'm worried
about being restricted to the foods on the Quick
Weight Loss Diet. That's because I've learned the
body is a very complicated mechanism with a wide
variety of chemical components as this shows." She
handed me a newspaper clipping containing this statement:

The body of a person weighing 140 pounds contains the following chemicals:

enough fat for seven cakes of soap . . .
enough carbon for 9,000 pencils . . .
enough phosphorus to make 2,200 match
heads . . .
enough magnesium for a dose of salts . . .
enough iron for a medium-size nail . . .
enough lime for whitewashing a doghouse . . .
enough sulphur to rid one dog of fleas . . .
enough water to fill a gallon jug.

I returned the clipping and suggested to her, "Paste
this clipping in your scrapbook along with the snap-
shots that will keep reminding you how terribly overweight and misshapen you were. You stay with my
diet and let me worry about the chemical composition
of your body. That's my job." Fortunately she put aside
her fears and lost weight rapidly.

Beware of Saying, "I Eat Like a Bird." Whenever a
patient tells me this, I point out that the problem here
usually is definitely "eating like a bird." A bird does
not generally eat much at a time. He pecks a little
here and a little there. By the end of each day he
has eaten quite a peck of food. That "pecking" by
humans all day or all evening or both can add up to
an awful lot of calories.

At my suggestion, a worried wife kept track of an
evening's accumulation of calories by her overweight
husband. He complained constantly that he was gaining weight even though "I eat like a bird, practically
nothing all day long." She kept a running listing of
what he ate in a peck here and a peck there during
the course of an evening of reading the newspapers,
chatting a while and watching television.

When she added up the calories "per peck," the
total came to over 2,000 calories! Her spouse didn't
believe it until she showed him the listing and the
figures in black and white. He later lost weight rapid-

ly on the Quick Weight Loss Diet which doesn't permit such "peckings" of high-calorie snacks.

Make a Low-Calorie Checklist. There is a tendency for formerly overweight individuals on Stay Slim Eating to say now and then, "I just don't know what to eat. Nothing appeals to me." The problem is usually lazy thinking or a lack of imagination. You may find this little trick helpful:

Go through the pages of food listings in this book and put a checkmark alongside each food you like which is low in calories. Then, whenever you find yourself saying, "I don't know what to eat," open the book. Go through your checklist. You're sure to find plenty that appeals to you and will satisfy you most at that particular time.

Dieting With High Blood Pressure: One of my patients, a noted scientist in a field outside of medicine, was fearful of going on the high protein Quick Weight Loss Diet because he was 30 percent overweight and had a high blood pressure of 180/100. From his "scientific viewpoint," he figured that the burning up of his own body fat was equivalent to going on a high saturated fatty acid diet similar to eating butter, cream and animal fats.

Using some technical terms necessarily, the answer went like this: Obesity and high blood pressure are very dangerous. Obesity without high blood pressure is dangerous. While it is so that the body will convert its own fat into cholesterol, it is also true that a low fat diet (exogenous) or your own body fat (endogenous), will not raise the cholesterol of the blood. The body can and does produce 150 to 170 milligrams of cholesterol even if no fat is eaten. Also, the body maintains a blood sugar of 80 to 120 milligrams whether little or no carbohydrates are eaten.

Experiments have shown that eating a great deal of fat produces excess cholesterol. Eating unsaturated fatty acids instead may reduce it. However, if you keep on eating large amounts of non-saturated oils, you still will have high cholesterol.

Overweight produces a fatty, "creamy" blood. When you burn up your own fat, you may increase the amount of triglycerides in the blood, but this has not been shown to produce arteriosclerosis (thickening and hardening of the arteries). In reducing, it is more important as the primary goal to lose weight than to aim at reducing the cholesterol. Invariably the blood presure will come down as your weight goes down to normal—and your life expectancy will be normal.

In summary, if you go on the QWL Diet, your cholesterol and the fatty acids in the blood will *not* be increased but will either remain normal or be lessened.

Is Quick Reducing Desirable? This question keeps coming up. I have answered it various times in this book but reemphasis may be necessary. My basic, *proved* answer is that among the thousands of my patients who have lost weight by quick-reducing methods, not one has developed any irreversible symptoms or diseases. All have looked better and felt better upon achieving ideal weight; this includes celebrated actors and actresses, musicians, composers, producers, doctors, scores of doctors' wives, many nurses, nutritionists, professors, and others.

Some patients brought up the fact that the Council on Foods and Nutrition of the American Medical Association has expressed the opinion that quick weight loss or large fluctuations may be harmful. I pointed out that if the Council believed this for certain, the ambiguous term "may be" would not be used. Some doctors, "nutritionists," and others have been crying "wolf" for many years, but to date have not been able to show any harmful effects from sound quick reducing methods as recommended here.

Of course, a diet that has no vitamin C will produce

scurvy eventually. If a diet has no vitamin B, it will produce beriberi. If it has no calcium, it will produce rickets or soft bones. If it has no protein, it will produce other types of disease. But this is assuming that it will be a *permanent* diet, not just for weeks or months but for years. Nowhere do I advocate such permanency.

With the Quick Weight Loss Diet and other quick reducing diets, I have stated repeatedly that vitamin tablets or other available forms are to be taken daily to guard against deficiencies (which probably would not occur). In cases of gout or other diseases, I have stated emphatically that such dieting should be done under a physician's care. For the otherwise healthy woman or man, these quick reducing methods are essential lifesavers to get weight off and keep it off.

Use the QWL Diet Again and Again. Please keep in mind from now on that I developed the Stillman Quick Weight Loss Diet as a method which will stand you in good stead whenever the occasion may arise that you must once again lose weight. You will have learned, like thousands of my patients, that it is very simple and easy to go back on the QWL Diet and *immediately* start losing the extra pounds.

Keeping your weight down permanently is a question of sustained willpower. The practical fact is that if a method of reducing takes too long, the average individual will soon lose hope, will be discouraged and will stay fat. You must be taught a method which is not only rapid but is easily repeated. This is it.

Day of Deprivation. Many of my patients have found it surprisingly easy to set aside a "day of deprivation" each week. On that day they eat no solid food, just drink quantities of water and other non-caloric liquids, and take a couple of vitamin tablets. By limiting the fasting to just one day they find it easier to stay slim.

They say invariably that they feel better the next day. Instead of eating more the day after fasting they find they're eating less and losing weight more rapidly.

Stop at Ideal Weight. When you've reached your ideal weight, don't try to lose more pounds just to prove to yourself and others that you can. When I told a patient that she should indulge a little more rather than lose more weight, she answered, "My dress size should be 12 but until this week I could only wear 18, then 16, then 14 and finally 12, now. But I want to tell my friends I'm wearing a size 8!" I advised against this. It's healthier to be a little underweight than over-weight. However, I recommend the happy medium—*ideal weight*—for feeling and looking your best.

11. ANSWERS TO DIETERS'
COMMON EXCUSES

You now have all the instructions you need for losing weight *successfully*, as so many in my care have done. I have found it has helped patients to give them in advance the answers to common excuses that I've heard innumerable times from overweights who are hesitant to diet or who are faltering. The facts are stated here in straight, common sense doctor-to-patient terms, as in my office. I hope you'll read them carefully, as they can help you achieve the healthful, attractive slimness you want.

> *"I heard that somebody died from dieting,*
> *so I'm going to stop my diet."*

(One woman made this excuse after Quick Loss dieting had reduced her from 201 pounds to 146, and was headed for her ideal weight of 135.) In my entire experience no one in my care has ever become seriously ill from dieting, let alone worse than when overweight. When I've looked into other reported instances I've always found that dieting itself was never the cause. (She went on with her dieting and is now lovely and healthy at her desired weight, years later.)

> *"I felt fatigued so I ate and broke my diet."*

In the great majority of cases a person doesn't eat because he's fatigued. He simply uses this as an excuse. I checked this patient thoroughly and said, "There's no physical reason for you to feel tired all the time. Conditioning and environment have taught you to reach for something to eat without a reason, often even without hunger. Others will drink or smoke too much or chew their nails. You think that food in the stomach is the answer to tiredness so you use fatigue as an excuse to stuff yourself. If you'll fully recognize that it's an excuse and not a real bodily need you'll stop making the excuse and stop excess eating accordingly." (He thought about it and went on dieting without any further "feeling of fatigue.")

I also tell patients who complain of fatigue to move around more and get more exercise—a very helpful antidote to that tired feeling overweights often get from characteristic inactivity. I suggest these rules: "Don't lie down if you can sit. Don't sit if you can stand. Don't stand if you can walk." All this minor activity not only wakes you up and helps dispel fatigue but it also increases your expenditure of calories.

> *"I sprained my ankle, felt sorry for myself,*
> *so I ate to appease myself."*

I told her: "Not only were you lame due to your ankle but you gave yourself a lame excuse. There's no physical relationship between a sprained ankle and a fatty stomach except that overweight probably contributed to your awkwardness and caused the accident. You'll be less likely to have such accidents when you become slim and graceful. You'll have better balance and reflexes. It's far better treatment for a sprained ankle to lose weight fast than to gain more.

Another patient told me that she'd "read somewhere" that drinking lots of rich milk—forbidden on her Quick Weight Loss Diet—would help her broken leg to knit. So she was gulping milk and had gained back ten of the pounds she had lost. She was very vague about where she'd found such incorrect information. When she faced the fact that she was deluding herself she went back on the diet and lost weight rapidly.

"I had to go off the diet because I craved cookies."

Your answer to such an excuse is in the selection you have among over 60 diets in this book. You can't eat cookies on the Quick Loss Diet because the carbohydrates break up the efficient functioning of the method, as explained. You can switch to the temptation diet, indulge your craving for cookies and still lose weight, then return to the Quick Loss method and continue your rapid, steady weight loss. I've given you a diet for "cravers"—if necessary, use it.

"I ate when I wasn't supposed to because I had a 'hunger headache.'"

You'll find details about "hunger headaches" elsewhere but the vital point here is that you're kidding yourself with such an excuse. If your headache is genuinely due to hunger you can satisfy it on the Quick Loss Diet by eating a hard-boiled egg or 2 tablespoons of cottage cheese or a chicken leg or a slice of lean meat or fish. "Realize this," I told this patient, "and next time get rid of the headache, which probably won't even occur, by eating something that's on your diet instead of a forbidden calorie-rich food."

"I lost 5 pounds on your Quick Loss Diet, then put it all back over a social weekend."

Very few of my patients break their diet by the end of the first week and I blame myself for not getting my instructions across so that this woman would have the needed strong motivation. She finally realized that she was losing her attractiveness and endangering her health, and that saving herself was a matter of staying on the Quick Loss Diet every day for weeks, not breaking down 52 weekends of the year. She gained the firm realization of what she must do. She told her hostesses and guests that she was reducing as a matter of self-respect and life-or-death so far as she was concerned. By strengthening her resolve and pride she reestablished the diet and went from 150 pounds to her desired weight of 115.

"I can't stick with my diet because of necessary heavy business luncheons."

There are two ways to answer this excuse. Many of my businessmen patients have simply told clients and associates at lunch that, "I'm slimming down for my health so I ask your indulgence. No reason for you not to eat what you want. In a few months I hope to be at my proper weight and in the best possible health. Then I won't have to be this strict."

The other way, also effective, is to choose the one meal a day diet. Don't overeat at lunch but eat normally enough so that the matter of dieting doesn't come up. That's your meal for the day. Have coffee and vitamins for breakfast, coffee and cottage cheese for dinner.

"My menstrual period was different from usual, I became frightened and had to eat."

If something is wrong with your menses, as I told this patient, then eating certainly isn't going to cure it. Instead of gulping a big meal or a load of sweets, thus cloaking your symptoms by appetite gratification, you should see your doctor. He'll tell you what is really the trouble and will act to correct the problem. Swallowing an ice cream soda isn't the solution.

When something hurts you or worries you, get the proper treatment from a doctor—not from a dish of ice cream. Breaking the diet won't solve a thing, it will only keep you from your goal of a slim, attractive, healthier body. (With this woman, her menstrual difficulty was quickly checked by administering a simple diuretic. She resumed Quick Loss dieting and stopped looking for relief from every problem by grabbing forbidden food. She has achieved her ideal weight and a beautiful figure, maintained for 3 years now.)

"I keep breaking my diet because my hostess piles food on my plate and I can't be ungracious so I eat it up."

There's no sin in leaving food on your plate as soon as you've eaten enough to stop your hunger. Put down your fork and don't pick it up again. "The easiest way to get rid of weight is to leave it on your plate." You're better off to stick with your diet and tell your hostess so *before* she piles up your plate. Anyone who would consider you "ungracious" for being firm about improving your health and appearance isn't a worthy friend. Don't cloak your own weakness and sense of self-indulgence by calling it graciousness or politeness. Be firm next time and watch your hostess respect you for it.

"I get too irritable, depressed and mean when dieting, so I have to eat whatever my stomach craves."

It's a weak excuse to blame irritability and depression on your stomach's cravings. You're evading the real reasons which may include idleness, unhappiness with your appearance and way of life. The fatter you get, the worse off you are. Get on the move, get interested in stimulating things as suggested on other pages. Treat your mind instead of your stomach. Success at becoming thin has improved the entire outlook of many of my patients.

"I can't go on a diet because I have ulcer-like pains in my stomach so I keep drinking milk all day and putting on weight."

(I've heard this from many people who were not my patients but whom I've encountered socially.) If you have "ulcer-like pains" then you either have an ulcer or think you have. You should see a doctor immediately instead of pouring in milk on top of your other food. The correct diet will counteract hyperacidity in the stomach. If you are overweight, the doctor may very likely put you on a reducing diet which permits you 6 glasses of skim milk and 6 bananas a day and nothing else, alternated every other hour.

"My mother was sick so I ate to drown my troubles."

This is one of the most common and sickest excuses of all, that, for one reason or another, "I ate to drown my troubles." Of course your emotional anxiety is very real. Overeating is one of the worst ways to treat it. Overeating when you're overweight especially drowns your heart and lungs, clogs your arteries and shortens your life. If you wish to serve and help your mother (or solve other problems that produce emotional tension and anxiety) don't injure yourself by overeating. Then you may not be able to help because you've developed your own infirmities. Instead, direct your thoughts and energies into painting, writing, knitting, sewing or other productive pursuits.

"I developed canker sores from dieting so I had to eat."

It's possible for allergic patients to develop canker sores from foods, but upon questioning this patient further I learned that she had had canker sores quite a few times *before* she started dieting. She had honestly had a complete lapse of memory about the previous times. Convinced that there was no relationship, she went back on her diet.

I can't begin to list all the ills and symptoms that patients attribute to dieting until they are reminded that they have experienced the same troubles long before. One woman claimed that she'd developed "a lump in the throat" due to dieting. I diagnosed this as *globus* (ball) *hystericus* (emotional) which is a common symptom among nervous and tense individuals. She admitted that she'd had it in the past quite often. After her mind was relieved by understanding the cause, I told her to indulge in eating her favorite foods for a few days, then return to her Quick Loss Diet. Instead, her "lump in the throat" vanished at once; she returned to dieting immediately and stuck with it. Once slimmed down she was much less nervous and tense.

"I was so bored that I ate and broke my diet."

These cases are sad and all too common. I urge all such patients to become interested in some activity. In my practice, and in talking with people, I find that many heavy women eat because they haven't much else to occupy their time or mental and physical energies. There are exceptions, of course. By and large I've noted that older women with lessened responsibilities tend to be heaviest. Busy housewives occupied with children and community activities are more likely to be only slightly overweight. Alert career women and secretaries on the go are slimmer on the average. It helps you stay on a diet and then on effective Stay Slim Eating if you keep yourself busy, interested, active, on the move.

"I had a sore throat so I took lots of honey and ice cream to soothe it."

Don't demean yourself by using such an obviously

weak excuse, treating your throat (or other ills) with doubtful or useless weight-producing "remedies." A sore throat needs bed rest and proper medication, not rich sweets that make your already overworked, fat-laden organs work harder than ever and pull down your overall health. Another patient told me that he had a sore tooth so he could only eat rich, creamy cereals, ice cream and malteds. I told him to see a dentist and to switch to the temptation diet. After a few days he called me apologetically and said he was back on the Quick Loss Diet and losing weight rapidly; he didn't fall off again.

"I developed polio and was confined to bed and house for a long time without moving around so I gained weight terribly."

I told this person whom I met socially: "It's too bad that you weren't instructed to eat very little. Since your expenditure of energy was so small, you needed very little food to supply your body's requirements. It happens to so many people, not ill, who cut down on their activity without cutting down on food intake. The only alternative to weight gain when there is a lack of activity and exercise is to eat less." (The polio victim, with her strong will, went on the Quick Loss Diet and lost her excess weight rapidly. This was particularly important and helpful for her since over-weight was further inhibiting her freedom of movement.)

"I went to Europe, ate too much, and became very fat."

Can one really blame a trip to Europe for his own self-indulgence? Another of my overweight patients went to Europe and came back slimmer than when she left. She and her husband were absorbed by everything they saw and did. Their activity was increased by going to museums and places of interest, collecting antiques, working off a lot of energy (and calories). They ate in the famous restaurants, enjoying the food thoroughly without overeating. They were aware that stuffing themselves could only add fat to their bodies and take away years of life. I urge you to slim down and watch your eating wherever you go so that you can stay healthy and enjoy a long, vigorous life.

"The skin on my neck was sagging so I tried to fill it out by eating."

Except for the very aged the natural elasticity of the skin will bring it back to normal soon when reducing, if it sags at all. If you're youthful this is no problem, so by all means reduce fast and early to avoid this temporary condition ever. In any case, at any age, be patient and your skin will return to normal. If you're quite elderly you'll feel in so much better health when slim that you won't mind wrinkling or sagging if it should occur.

"I've been a bad girl, I ate like mad."

There are many crimes that are much worse. You're not the first one to slip off a diet, especially if you're on a balanced, gradual diet. Start over again. This time pick the Quick Weight Loss Diet or another quick action diet that suits you best. Each time you go back on a diet (if you slip off) it becomes easier to stay on it and lose weight rapidly. Use your mental energy to stay on the diet instead of using it up in scolding yourself. By prodding yourself you can attain that slim figure which earns admiring (and envious) glances.

"After giving birth to my baby I wasn't able to take off the weight I gained. I couldn't stay on the diet."

Especially if you were slim before having your baby

(or at any weight), you can be just as slim afterward unless your doctor has given you any reason otherwise. Any change affecting your weight is extremely rare. It's just as important to you and your happy married life (often even more essential) to stay slim and attractive. Once your body has recovered fully from giving birth, the dieting recommendations given here should work for you. This is true no matter how many times you may have given birth. If you overeat, don't blame your baby for your own unwarranted self-indulgence.

> *"I felt that I was getting anemic and developing 'tired blood' on the diet, so I quit."*

I advised this gentleman that he was developing "tired blood" only in his overactive imagination. Blood tests proved conclusively that he was not "getting anemic." Being a sensible businessman who believed the specific results of the tests, he went back to quick loss dieting. He phoned me a week later to say that instead of feeling tired he was enjoying a sense of extra vigor and buoyancy due to shedding excess, burdensome fat.

> *"Subconsciously I believe that I hate my mother, so I keep eating to stay fat and unattractive just to spite her."*

I didn't laugh at this because I hear that kind of thing very often from overweights. Such excuses are very popular today with self-psychoanalysts who grab at any reason to keep stuffing themselves. Usually such "psychological anxiety" alibis are claptrap. Psychiatric problems should be treated by a psychiatrist, not by yourself, and certainly not by well-meaning but misled friends. I urged this patient to put aside thoughts of her relationship to her mother (at least as it influenced her eating) and to try the Quick Weight

Loss Diet for one week. She was so pleased at losing nine pounds that week that nothing could have stopped her from continuing to reduce down to her ideal weight. In a later visit she told me, "I love my figure and my mother."

"I broke my diet with candy because suddenly I needed something sweet."

Eating "something sweet" today doesn't mean breaking your diet. A satisfying "sweet" can be a glass of refreshing non-caloric beverage. You can also enjoy tea or black coffee with artificial sweetening. You can have handy some artificially sweetened little mints in convenient rolls, non-sugar chewing gum and artificially sweetened gumdrops to satisfy your sweet tooth without adding calories. However, don't gorge yourself on them.

"I ate because I had cramps in my legs from dieting, and heard that unless I ate a lot I would get a floating kidney, a hernia or varicose veins."

All this is utter nonsense yet I've heard such alibis again and again. I assure my patient that whoever told him this probably wanted him to stay heavy. The fact is that the skin and muscles tighten where the fat is lost. One of the best treatments for varicose veins is losing excess fat. It also helps relieve cramps in the legs and arthritis of the knee, ankle and foot.

"Since I started taking 'birth control pills,' I've found myself overeating and putting on more weight."

I convinced this patient that she'd only given birth to another excuse to indulge herself, since there was no valid reason why "birth control pills" should cause her to overeat. (However, occasionally some women seem to retain a little extra fluid when first starting

on the contraceptive pills.) Such medication contains
no calories and does not act physiologically to increase
the appetite. She protested weakly, "A friend told me
that these pills make a person eat more." Once she
realized that such pills have as little relation to the
appetite as aspirin, she returned to her Stay Slim Eating, along with occasional weeks on quick loss dieting. She then kept her weight down and her figure
lovely.

*"I'm already 15 pounds overweight so I decided
'what's the difference if I add a few more pounds'—
and I let myself go."*

I told this patient that each individual's system has
its breaking point and that adding "a few more
pounds" or even one more pound may be just enough
extra burden to bring on serious illness and disability.
Every pound of excess fat taken off lessens such danger. She was persuaded, like many others, to think
positively instead of negatively. Instead of letting "a
few more pounds" pile on, her daily goal—like a game
—was transformed into seeing "a few more pounds"
vanish from the scale. On the Quick Weight Loss Diet
she was able to see this positive result with her own
eyes in the scale's "numbers game" day after day. As
her weight went down her spirits went up. She has
become slender and attractive, and has been married.
Whenever she sees "a few more pounds" show on the
scale she returns to the Quick Weight Loss Diet for a
week or so.

*"I break my diet at bedtime because I can't fall asleep
unless I have a glass of milk and a sandwich
or cakes and cookies."*

This patient had convinced himself that only those
fattening snacks could put him to sleep. He promised
me that for the next week he'd substitute a moderate

portion of cottage cheese and a non-caloric beverage as his bedtime treat. After three days he phoned to say that he'd enjoyed a full, sound sleep the night before. By the end of the week he'd stopped eating *anything* at bedtime and was sleeping well. Since then he has taken off most of the excess weight which was crowding his organs and preventing healthful, comfortable sleep. He's had no trouble with insomnia at ideal weight.

"I was operated on for gallstones, put on a great deal of weight and haven't been able to stick to a diet and take it off."

This woman was trying to reduce by cutting down on her eating gradually since she feared bad effects from a stringent diet. She'd heard that it's healthiest to eat a lot after recuperating from an operation, which is exactly wrong. I reassured her that she'd recovered fully, and put her on the Quick Weight Loss Diet. Within 10 weeks she took off 30 pounds. She then went on Stay Slim Eating for a month. She returned to quick loss dieting and soon took off 10 more pounds which brought her down to her ideal weight and figure. She realizes now that it was excess fat which caused her weakness after recovering from the operation, and that effective dieting brought back her strength as well as attractive appearance.

"My conscience troubles me if I leave good food on my plate or throw it out, so I overeat."

I say to such patients, "Please realize that one of the worst things you can do to yourself in your overweight condition is to stuff your system and add dangerous pounds. It becomes easy to convince your 'conscience' if you're once convinced of this fact: The food you leave on your plate or throw out can't kill you; overeating it can."

*"I was so dry all week I kept gulping sodas
and up went my weight."*

Reach for all the sweet sodas you want but next
time make sure that they're non-caloric. You can drink
5 or more refreshing bottles a day and add practically
no calories instead of over 500 calories daily from
sugary drinks. There's no difference in taste.

*"If I do anything wrong, I punish myself
by overeating."*

My answer to this woman was: "The fact that you
recognize this common flimsy excuse as your own is
encouraging. You're not the first to slip off a diet. But
by overeating, you're only doing something else wrong
to your looks and your health, so you would have to
punish yourself for overeating by more overeating.
That's a silly, stupid cycle that you can certainly
break. If you do anything wrong, or if anything goes
wrong, you can cope with it better if you're healthier
and more vigorous and alert than if you're burdened
with fat and lethargic in mind and body. By following
the Quick Loss Diet you'll be better equipped mentally
and physically to cope with whatever goes wrong."

*"I felt uncomfortable because I was constipated
so I ate a lot."*

Constipation and lack of bowel movement can happen on any diet which doesn't contain much waste material. The Quick Loss method, also the formula, high
fat and high protein, and fasting diets, for example,
have very little residue so that a bowel movement is
delayed. You may not have a movement for a week.
Don't be concerned, because your worries are strictly
psychological. A person can go up to 4 weeks without
a bowel movement and suffer no ill effects. If you're
concerned, take a mild laxative such as milk of magnesia or mineral oil.

*"I can't afford to reduce because I have to look
robust and prosperous in my business, not sickly
and skinny like a dieter."*

I heard this excuse from a friend at lunch whom
I'd warned about his alarmingly increasing overweight. Then he belched and grumbled, "I'm full of
gas. I have an important meeting at 2:30 and I'm worried about it." I asked him, "Do I look sickly and
skinny?" He said, "No, you're an exception." I insisted,
"I'm not an exception. You're using an empty, fake
excuse to justify your overindulgence and weakness of
will. I want you to lose weight starting tomorrow, because I don't want to lose you before your time."

*"So I'm 40 pounds overweight but I'm the picture of
health. I can lift my weight in wildcats and lick them
too. No reason for me to reduce and become a skinny
weakling. Besides, I've always been heavy and it
hasn't hurt me."*

Sad to relate, this "picture of health," in his early
40's, was felled by a fatal heart attack one week after
he told me this at a dinner party. Despite old-fashioned
notions that still persist, weight gain leads to weakness,
not strength. If you don't believe me, believe the death
statistics and start getting down to your ideal weight
right now. Whether or not you've "always been heavy,"
overweight is dangerous and harmful. The sooner you
realize this and start reducing, the better your chances
for a healthy, longer life.

You've heard hundreds of other excuses like these
and so have I. Each empty excuse is another way of
saying that stuffing oneself with excessive, calorie-rich
foods is more important than vigorous health, attractive appearance and life itself. As far back as the
1600's, Gabriel Meurier put it this way:

"He who excuses himself accuses himself."

12. FACTS TO HELP "SCARE" THE FAT OFF YOU

I consider overweight the nation's No. 1 health problem. It impairs and kills more people than any other sickness. I believe it is vital to publish these proved facts because, shocking as it is, most overweights must *diet or die younger*.

When Dr. Louis M. Orr was president of the American Medical Association, he was asked in a newspaper interview, "Do you consider cancer the greatest threat we face?" He answered, "No. Cancer is the most dreaded disease in the United States. But the greatest danger to the health of the American people is obesity."

If you are overweight and have any doubts about the importance and urgency of starting your Quick Loss dieting *now*, the facts here may convince you once and for all. The following Death Chart is based on a number of expert estimates. Some are higher, some lower, but these figures are generally agreed upon:

DEATH CHART FROM OVERWEIGHT

If you are overweight, you will die younger, according to statistics. You will shorten your life by one to ten years or more, depending on how much excess fat you carry. It is conservatively estimated that 25% of men in their thirties and 35% of men in their fifties are about 20 pounds overweight. They are cut down before their life expectancy by heart disease, strokes, emphysema (shortness of breath, difficulty in breathing), diabetes and many other afflictions. The following averages apply to men and women:

10% overweight 10%	shorter life span
20% overweight 20%	"
30% overweight 30%	"
40% overweight 40%	"
50% or more overweight..............50% to 200%	"

In other words, if you're 10% overweight, your chances of dying earlier than your average life expectancy are 10% higher. If your ideal weight is 160 pounds, and if your normal life expectancy is age 70, you're likely to die at age 63. You'll lose 7 years of living. In effect, you will have committed suicide at age 63. The more overweight you are, the more years you're wiping out.

Those are the frightening odds you're gambling with on your own life. Expert figures vary, as noted, but all agree that the more excess weight you carry, the more you invite earlier death.

If you're 10% or more heavier than your ideal weight, then you should consider yourself an "overweight" taking years off your life. Looking at it another way, you're making yourself look and feel years older than you really are. Your organs are aging too fast for your years.

Even small increases in weight lower your life expectancy. If you're 5% heavier than your ideal weight, you're not fat. But for health's sake, as well as improved appearance, you're much better off losing the few extra pounds and maintaining your ideal weight or slightly under.

SICKNESS IN OVERWEIGHTS

The following is from a publication by the American Medical Association, warning about the dangers of overweight:

You're a Fatty if you weigh 10 to 15 percent more than your desirable weight. If you're supposed to weigh in around 130–140, and you're pushing 160, then you're one of the 34 million Americans who is overweight.

What Do a Few Extra Pounds Mean? It could be the difference between good and bad health. In some cases, you're actually killing yourself by staying fat. Insurance companies can easily prove:

High blood pressure is found twice as frequently in fatties.

Hardening of the arteries is three times as much in the obese.

Diabetes and *arthritis* are somewhat more common diseases of those pleasingly plump.

The overweight are *poorer marginal risks.*

Serious heart disorders and *strokes* are more prevalent in the obese.

If you're not sufficiently impressed yet with the seriousness of overweight as a death hazard, consider also how it makes living far less pleasant. Even the famed French gourmet, Brillat-Savarin, warned: "Well, go ahead and eat and grow fat, become ugly, heavy, have asthmatic attacks and die choked by your own fat."

Overweights are more susceptible to many common and even minor diseases. They have less resistance to infection. They have more accidents than slim people. In my practice, fat persons were far more afflicted with worse and longer-lasting colds than those at ideal weight. They also complained of many more general vague "miseries" which prevented or reduced the daily pleasures of living.

A medical newsletter states: "Life Insurance companies have placed obesity high on the list of conditions which will considerably shorten life. The overweight person not only will not live as long as others, but he or she will also be a more frequent sufferer from fatigue, various bodily discomforts and malfunctions, and even serious and often crippling diseases such as diabetes, arteriosclerosis (hardening of the arteries), and certain cardiac conditions. (Obesity is the condition of being overweight when it reaches 10–20% over normal weight.)"

Another medical report: "Overweight produces a 2½ times greater risk of coronary (heart) trouble than normal weight."

Dermatologists warn that obesity promotes and accelerates a variety of skin disorders and accompanying undesirable symptoms.

EXCESS FAT SPURS BODY MALFORMATION

The top illustrations show how an ideal weight figure (left) is actually bent out of shape by excess weight (right), straining the muscles, body structure and organs at many points.

HOW OVERWEIGHT SPURS FOOT, LEG AND BACK ILLS

The lower left illustration on page 194 shows how the weight of the body normally bisects the knee cap and falls between the large toe and second toe. Excessive overweight (lower right illustration) usually throws the feet outward. Weight does not fall at midline as desirable, but beyond the knee cap and toward the back of the arch. This may produce severe osteoarthritis (bone arthritis) of the pelvis, knee and ankle joints, with severe flat feet, varicose veins and general fatigue.

THE INSIDE STORY OF OVERWEIGHT EFFECT ON ORGANS

The simplified drawings on page 196 indicate what

IDEAL WEIGHT   OVERWEIGHT

happens in a man 5′ 6″ tall, weighing 190 pounds instead of his ideal weight of 130–143.

The head and neck are enlarged due to fat deposits under the scalp skin and on the muscle layers. Fat depots all over the body demand increases of blood pumped by the heart.

The heart is covered with a layer of fat especially at the top. This is very burdensome to its proper functioning. The heart is pushed up into the neck and also brought forward. If you placed your fingers between the two collar bones, you would feel distinct pulsations, normally not apparent.

The main blood vessels are enlarged in order to carry blood to the excessive amount of fat deposited in the arms and chest wall.

Lung capacity is reduced at least one-third because of crowding by fat. The liver is enlarged to 1½ times its original size and is pushed up into the lung cage. The stomach is ballooned up to three times its normal size and pushes up into the chest. The abdomen is raised high because of the tremendous amount of fat in the abdominal cavity (a very large tumor or a large pregnancy acts similarly).

The coronary blood vessels cannot enlarge yet they must carry the same amount of blood to the heart muscle. If the rate of flow is increased by extra work or emotion or a huge meal, the heart cries out that the heart muscles are being undernourished because of scant supplies of available blood. In the picture at the right, note that there is plenty of breathing space and the heart does not reach up into the neck as at the left.

DANGERS FROM OVERSTUFFING WITH A HUGE MEAL

What happens when you're overweight and are overstuffed by a tremendous meal? The huge ballooning stomach starts pressing and irritating the dome of the

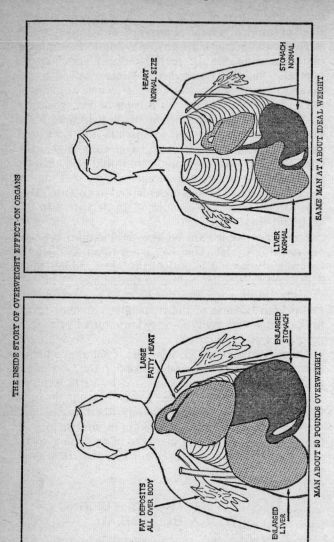

THE INSIDE STORY OF OVERWEIGHT EFFECT ON ORGANS

LARGE FATTY HEART

FAT DEPOSITS ALL OVER BODY

ENLARGED STOMACH

ENLARGED LIVER

MAN ABOUT 50 POUNDS OVERWEIGHT

HEART NORMAL SIZE

STOMACH NORMAL

LIVER NORMAL

SAME MAN AT ABOUT IDEAL WEIGHT

diaphragm, often resulting in belching and hiccuping. The pressure is continued upward and impedes the action of the heart, moving it into a more horizontal position and making it more difficult for the coronary arteries to be filled with needed blood.

The upward pressures of the stomach and heart narrow the breathing space of the lungs so that the person's breathing is heavy and labored. Liver and intestinal juices are poured out by the gallon. Eventually, with such excesses, the liver is likely to become fatty. The bile thickens. The pancreas may exhaust its power to produce not only juices for digestion, but also its supply of insulin.

As the excessively heavy meal is absorbed, the fat ingested reaches the blood vessels in such quantity that the blood becomes thick and "creamy." Its motion is slowed. Then the blood may clot at the junction of the arteries, possibly producing either a coronary thrombosis or a cerebral thrombosis (coagulation). The fat may be deposited in the very small arteries. With repetition, the accumulations of fat may eventually clog and block the arteries.

If one eats too much over a long period, the liver which normally provides a clearing factor is damaged. The fat remains in the blood for a much longer time. This tends again to produce dreaded arteriosclerosis (hardening of the arteries).

SURGERY PROBLEMS, FATIGUE AFFLICT OVERWEIGHTS

Surgery is far more hazardous for those carrying excess layers of fat. Preparing a fat person for surgery, the anesthetist is more concerned. The surgeon must worry as he cuts through pounds and layers of fat. Even the wounds of the fat heal more slowly. Many times the surgeon will postpone surgery if the operation is not an emergency and send a fat patient back to the doctor to be reduced first.

Not the least of the common, everyday afflictions of most overweight individuals is chronic fatigue and a tired, dragged-out, lethargic feeling which may interfere with normal sex life as well as other aspects of daily living.

If you need any further proof that overweight is a real and ever-present danger to the individual, realize that life insurance companies are cautious in issuing policies to fat people and often charge them higher rates. Such extra charges are then reduced to normal if the individual reduces and maintains his ideal weight. It even pays in dollars and cents here to slim down.

I've touched only superficially on the harm excess weight can do to the heart, blood vessels and other organs. My purpose is to jolt you into starting to reduce now if you're overweight.

YOUR BALL-AND-CHAIN OF FAT

If you're 20 pounds overweight, for instance, you're dragging a terribly burdensome ball-and-chain of fat behind you with every step you take. That unrelenting weight is pulling on your heart and entire system. Even when you stand still, sit or lie down, your heart and organs must support that 20-pound ball-and-chain. To stop being a prisoner of that ever-present, debilitating load, start a successful quick reducing program now.

LIFE OR DEATH? IT'S UP TO YOU

Yes, you can mention a number of overweight people who live to age 70, 80 and over, and who say, "Being fat didn't keep me from living to a ripe old age." Also, granted that there are some fatties who seem to be bubbling with energy—these are the rare exceptions. The facts prove that the odds are against long life or average life expectancy if you're overweight. Face it, as a whole, fat people die younger. Every time I see a grossly overweight person, I want to speak a warning: "Get that weight off, you're heading for an earlier death. Reduce and save your life!"

Don't try to excuse yourself, as many do, by claiming that, "Most of my excess weight is muscle, I'm not really fat." Overweight is overweight whether it's muscular or fatty. The fatty kind is more injurious but excess weight of any kind is a dangerous drag on a heart that has to pump extra blood and carry the extra load. Few overmuscled individuals are noted for longevity.

Many heavy patients have reported that afflictions they've suffered for years—backaches, headaches, gastric upsets, breathing difficulties and other ills—have vanished along with excess weight. You'll enjoy many blessings when you've rid yourself of that extra load of 10 or more pounds of burdensome fat. But don't consider yourself free of all ills automatically; slimming is not a cure-all. Have your doctor give you a complete checkup to make sure that you're in excellent condition all over.

Keep in mind always that calories count and can kill; but just counting calories won't help. Only reducing your calorie intake drastically and effectively will cause you to lose weight rapidly. The Quick Weight Loss Diet will take off that excess fat quickly and give you a new lease on a healthier life, a better chance for a happier life.

"HOW DEAR IS LIFE TO YOU?"

"The answer to the question for the individual is that life is priceless. To the family its loss is a major tragedy."

That statement in relation to the importance of proper health care was made by Dr. Willard C. Rappleye, Dean Emeritus of the Faculty of Medicine, Columbia University. I suggest that you ask yourself right now, "How dear is my life to my family and me?"

If you're overweight, particularly if you're considerably overweight, you're not holding life very dear. Even if life may not be priceless to you, realize that your loss would be a major tragedy to your family. Unless you get rid of that excess weight and slim down to your ideal weight, you're hastening your death. The preceding plain facts and many others prove it beyond question.

Unfortunately, the warnings and recommendations of preventive medicine are little heeded by most people. When a fat man or woman is told to reduce to lessen the danger of a heart attack or other serious damage, he or she usually waits until stricken and near death before taking the weight off.

Even then many victims start loading on the excess fat once more after they're up and about for a while. Perhaps the facts here will convince you to begin the Quick Weight Loss Diet or other effective reducing diets now.

There's grim humor in the statement by a commentator that "Things tend to even up—the more bodily weight you carry around, the shorter time you'll likely have to carry it." An old proverb tells that "Overeating destroys more than hunger." It destroys health and life itself.

Centuries ago, Hippocrates warned in his 44th Aphorism, "People who are fat are apt to die earlier than those who are slender." Centuries later "fat people" haven't learned to accept this, often because they think there's little hope of success in reducing. My recommendations here have helped others who had failed in their efforts before. Hopefully my methods will help you succeed where your previous attempts didn't.

On the other hand, if you never have decided and tried to take off burdensome excess weight, I trust that you'll start at once. Saying "I'm only 10 percent overweight, I'm not a fatty" is not a valid excuse. Once you

start to let yourself go the danger increases of undesirable, unbecoming fat piling on.

Recently a beautiful young woman whom I had
helped to become slim and who had stayed that way,
told me how she had finally managed to get her husband to reduce. "During our 12 years of married life,"
she said, "I couldn't get George to take off the fat
that was turning a handsome man into an uglier one
each year. He kept putting on weight until he scaled
over 240 pounds instead of the normal 175 pounds he
was when I married him. I tried to get him to visit you
or at least go on your diet, but he refused. He always
answered, 'I'm a happy fat man.'"

She shook her head. "I almost gave up. Last summer we rented a house at the beach. Most of the time
George wouldn't get into his swim trunks even though
he loves to swim. The few times he did go swimming
he looked like a tremendous beach ball with legs. No
one would ever know that there was a very handsome,
tall, thin man hiding inside that ugly mass of flab.

"It didn't help when I told him again and again
that I was afraid of his premature death because of
his shortness of breath and other evidences of deterio-
rating health. Finally I said straight out, 'George, I'm
ashamed of the way you look. I'm beginning to dis-
like being with you. Either you start slimming down
or I'm afraid that I'll eventually get to the point where
I'll have to leave you!'"

She beamed. "It worked. He couldn't get upset about
dying before his time. But this blow to his vanity, and
even suggesting that his overweight might be repulsive
to me, as well as to others, and could break up our
marriage—that did the trick. He made a deal with
me that he'd go on your Quick Weight Loss Diet for
just one short week. If he didn't lose weight—he
thought he was one of those people who couldn't—I
promised I'd shut up about it from then on.

"He's a man of his word. He stayed with the diet.
In that one short week he lost 17 pounds. Each morn-

ing he couldn't wait to step on the scale and shout to
me, 'Down three more pounds!'

"In two weeks he has dropped 26 pounds. He's starting to look young and handsome again. He's so thrilled
by the change, and how easily and pleasantly it happens on your method, that nothing can stop him now!"

This case fortunately has a happy ending. Too many
others I've known about have ended in family tragedy
with a woman leaving a grossly overweight husband
whom she couldn't stand to look at or live with any
more. More often the situation has been that of a man
leaving his overweight wife who had lost her figure,
her looks, her pride and spirit and finally her husband.

IT'S UP TO YOU

When I see an obese individual shoveling in the rich
food, my impulse is to snap at him, "Stop, you're dig-
ging your grave with your fork!" Of course I don't
speak out. It's not polite. It's not considered gracious
in our civilized society to tell someone that he's com-
mitting suicide by overeating. It's not "nice" to warn
a well-meaning woman that she's pushing her husband
into an early grave by overfeeding him.

As for the reactions of friends and acquaintances,
they're not going to tell you frankly that you're losing
your looks and your sex appeal by piling on ungainly
pounds. The only one that will tell you is your mirror,
and then only if you look at the reflected image clearly
and don't erase the unbecoming fat bulges with your
eyes.

I tell you specifically on these pages how to diet effectively. The proof that the method can work wonderfully is written in the tens of thousands of unwanted
pounds dropped by my patients. But neither I nor
anyone else can diet for you. I'm hopeful that you'll
start taking off weight determinedly now. Further,
that every time you may be tempted to stop dieting
and go back to putting on fat, you'll first re-read the

gruesome facts in this chapter and that they'll help keep you on your diet.

Remind yourself:

"I don't want to suffer from sickness and pain . . ."

"I don't want to be stricken by a heart attack brought on by self-indulgent overweight . . ."

"I don't want to die before my time because of gluttonous overeating . . ."

"I don't want to lose my looks under a blanket of lard and become an unpleasant sight, a misfit, seeming years older than I am . . ."

The means are here to start taking off excess weight now. As in the case of George, give yourself just one short week on the Quick Weight Loss Diet. See what wonderful things can start to happen for your health, your good looks, and your whole future.

13. IMPORTANT TIPS ON
DIETING PSYCHOLOGY

"The only thing we have to fear is fear itself," was the pivotal statement in the historic speech by President Franklin D. Roosevelt which started to turn the tide and pull Americans out of the doldrums of the great depression.

In my experience the principal psychological reason why so many overweights have failed to reduce is *fear*—fear of injury from dieting rather than fear of sickness and death from not dieting. The most damaging aspect of this ingrained deterrent is fear of losing weight too fast, of cutting down on food intake, of eating in a different manner.

Much of this fear is inculcated by the old-fashioned but still prevalent idea of mother scolding, "Eat! Eat! It's good for you!" Most all of us have been part of the scene of a child not hungry but mother exhorting, "Make yourself eat, otherwise you'll get weak and sick." The common wifely or motherly reaction, even today, "What? You had nothing to eat all day yesterday but a little broiled hamburger and lettuce on a diet? Are you trying to kill yourself? You'll get weak, you'll fall apart—eat! eat! eat!"

It's part of the general psychology about dieting that an all too common reaction about quick action dieting is, "I heard about that actress, what's-her-name, who went on a severe diet and died of starvation— and with all the money in the world and everything to live for. Terrible!" Or, "Who was that famous actor,

years ago, who had to get thin to play Hamlet and he
got sick and died? Not for me!"

This is all obvious nonsense, but it has been spouted
repeatedly by otherwise intelligent individuals who
can then devour their fattening foods with false self-
justification. Tracking down such cases invariably
proves that the persons, if they existed at all, were
mentally sick and died of a cause completely unrelated
to dieting. Furthermore such individuals, especially the
rich and famous, were under the care of physicians
who would have stopped any harmful dieting immediately.

WEAK EXCUSES FOR PERSONAL WEAKNESS

Clearly all these are just excuses not to diet, not to
break up one's cherished and indulgent eating habits,
not to deny oneself "the good things in life," even at
the risk of ill health and earlier death. I state repeatedly in this book that it's best to be checked by a
doctor before dieting, and certainly at any sign that
the diet may be harmful. The doctor's tests reveal
quickly whether any undesirable symptoms are physical or psychological disturbances.

I state again that if the self-denial involved in dieting results in mental or other illness, it is preferable
to stop dieting and stay fat. But I must reiterate conclusively that from my long and thorough experience
my quick action diets and instructions as detailed here
are safe, quick, effective life savers for the 95% of
people who have no metabolic or other serious disturbances. I have reduced thousands of men and
women who had failed in many previous attempts,
not only by giving them the effective quick loss dieting
techniques, but also by helping them to get rid of the
psychology of fear of quick weight loss.

Unfortunately some doctors and nutritionists contribute to and bolster the harmful psychological fears
by insisting that the only "proper" way to lose weight

is through "balanced dieting," "normal dieting methods" of eating a little less and cutting out a few high-calorie foods. Apparently it's not significant to them that such advice doesn't work for the overweights who try and fail, those who keep getting heavier and sicker from carrying burdensome fat.

To replace your own possible psychological fear of quick action dieting with a true and sound fear of not dieting and staying dangerously overweight, I urge you to read the proof to the contrary on these pages again and again. *Eat scared!*

THE RIGHT FRAME OF MIND FOR LOSING WEIGHT

You must develop a firm almost fanatic desire and resolve to lose dangerous excess weight; that's the reason for giving you the "Facts To Help 'Scare' The Fat Off You" (Chapter 12), and "Clearing Away False Fears About Quick-Reducing Diets" (Chapter 9). You must think, breathe, act and eat with the conviction that you'll achieve your target of reducing to healthful, ideal weight, and that you're getting nearer to the successful result every day.

It may be a little exasperating at first when you cut down on food you've become accustomed to like. You may feel the pangs of hunger for a few days. You may be tempted, but be sustained by the knowledge and certainty that *you're going to succeed this time*. You're going to realize sensibly that it's wasteful to worry about gaining back the weight you lose.

You must believe and keep reminding yourself constantly, that quick loss dieting techniques will cause you to get down to desired weight. Then you'll find that following effective Stay Slim Eating will help you stay thin from then on, with an assist from quick loss dieting as recommended whenever necessary. You're not just getting "empty advice" here, you're being given *methods that work*, and can work for you.

COMMON ALIBI: "EMOTIONAL FRUSTRATION"

You accomplish nothing by continuing to blame your present obesity on emotional frustration. I advise you to go on the Quick Weight Loss Diet or other of the quick action diets of your choice right now. You'll prove to yourself by the first week's dramatic drop in weight that you can reduce. That proof is your greatest prop in continuing the diet. I know that in a few weeks you'll feel much better and look much better. You'll find that you actually lose much of your desire for calorie-rich foods. You'll be delighted that you undertook this reducing program, and encouraged by the clear results, you'll stay with it until eventually you're as slim as you wish and should be.

Will you be crushed by a feeling of failure if, after losing quite a few pounds, you slip and start gaining again? No, not if you read again at that time, and time after time, the advice in this book. Realize that up-and-down reducing is neither uncommon nor harmful. Don't expect to succeed in a day; even when you hammer in a nail you can't do it with one blow, you must pound it again and again until it's firmly fixed.

By returning to the quick loss diet again, you'll lose again. And each dieting period results in lessening your desire for calorie-heavy foods. At the same time the sizable drop in poundage, accompanying personal gratification and compliments from others bolster your will to become thin. With each successive quick loss diet it becomes easier for most people to lose weight and keep taking off that excess fat.

When dieting, the warm, understanding, persistent encouragment of your doctor and your family and friends is very helpful. A cartoon noted a despairing fat lady being told by a salesman of bathroom scales, "As you step on it, it moans sympathetically." The most important encouragement you get from quick loss dieting is the sharp drop in numbers on the scale week after week and the slimmer image reflected by your mirror.

This is why the Quick Weight Loss Diet and other diets here are so helpful psychologically, as well as physically. This indisputable evidence that the diet is working and that your goal of a slim figure is not too far away often makes the difference between success or failure in sticking with your dieting resolve.

BE PROUD OF YOUR WILLPOWER

Dieting requires willpower on your part and you should be proud of yourself when you succeed. Cutting down on food, either gradually or suddenly (the latter is my usual recommendation), causes both physiological and psychological changes. If you're one of the minority who experiences "hunger headaches," fatigue or other undesirable symptoms, bear with them a few days and they'll usually go away. If they persist, see a doctor if it's only to have him tell you that there's nothing physically wrong. Usually the symptoms then vanish quickly and you're on the way to the sharp weight loss you want.

Be proud and be positive about your dieting. Don't act like a martyr or feel sorry for yourself. When you refuse desserts, second helpings or rich hors d'oeuvres at a party and others murmur, "You poor thing!"— speak up. Tell them that you're pleased to be dieting, that you're proud of the pounds you've lost to date and that you're determined to get right down to ideal weight. Every pound you take off and keep off is a small miracle worthy of self-congratulation.

Quote Jean Kerr's amusing line, "I feel about diets the way I feel about airplanes. They are wonderful things for other people to go on." Be proud that you're one of the "other people" who is accomplishing what every overweight would secretly like to. You're far stronger than the fatties who sigh, "I wish I could take off this weight, but I know that the only thing I'll lose will be the diet instructions." You're way ahead of them—you've stopped wishing, you're acting! The time is past when it was a status symbol to be fat in order to show prosperity; today the slim people are the ones who are envied.

DON'T OVERRATE THE VALUE OF FOOD

I've been amused by a cartoon showing two children impatiently waiting for food to be served at their mother's bridge party. One tells the other, "We'll eat soon. When they start talking about their diets they all get hungry." One thing that keeps many fat people that way is the psychological aspect of rating "good food" too highly in life.

I suggest that you regard high-calorie foods as your enemies. When you look at a piece of layer cake or other fattening delicacies, don't fail to see that "B-E-W-A-R-E" sign on it. If you find yourself weakening toward such temptations, reread "Facts To Scare The Fat Off You."

Keep these two points in mind. First, there are many things more important in life than stuffing yourself with the "finest foods" in the "finest restaurants," prepared by the "finest cook in town." There is appreciation of music, art, literature, your family and mostly your health and your longer life. Buy yourself a good book, an absorbing magazine; treat yourself to a movie, theater or concert with the money you'd have spent on rich foods. Feed your mind instead of your stomach for deeper enjoyment and lasting fulfillment.

Second, you can still be a gourmet by sampling or taking small portions of fine foods and really taking the time, eating very slowly, to appreciate their special flavors. The time will come when you can increase to moderate portions after you've finished your stringent dieting and are on Stay Slim Eating. The gains are certainly worth the sacrifice for the limited time it will take you to bring down your weight on the Quick Weight Loss Diet, for instance.

FACING BASIC INSECURITY

A funny, but somehow sad, line quoted to me was a wife asking her husband, "Be careful, this is a trick question. Did you love me more before I got fat?" This reflects the basic insecurity of most fat people who know underneath that they are less attractive physically and sexually, whether they admit it or not. Psychologically this is a corrosive influence, often souring and even spoiling many aspects of single and married life. Isn't it worth the sacrifice of denying yourself overindulgence in food in order to attain greater peace of mind and happiness for yourself and your loved ones?

It may also help keep you dieting to realize that you'll probably be saving money as you save calories. This point is sometimes a help psychologically, even to those who are quite wealthy.

Remember my previous advice—don't look dismally at the start into your future of weeks and perhaps months of dieting. There's an ancient saying that "a journey of a thousand miles begins with a single step." Concentrate on the first step and the next, not on the entire thousand miles. Keep telling yourself each morning after a look at the encouraging scale (if you haven't been cheating), "I will diet *one more day.*" Each day it becomes easier as your appetite diminishes with your decreasing weight.

Psychologically and calorie-wise it's good sense to keep busy at work, play, every possible interesting activity. Face it, you're breaking a pleasurable, entrenched habit when you deny yourself unlimited eating. Use every diversion you can. Many failures are due to idleness, boredom and nervousness which lead to the busy, compulsive habit of eating and swallowing, eating and swallowing.

DON'T KID YOURSELF WHEN DIETING

Losing weight isn't a breeze or a lighthearted matter, nor is it "kid stuff." Your health and length of life are at stake. So don't kid yourself that you're adhering to a diet if you're not. It helps many dieters psychologically to write down every item they eat so they don't fool themselves into saying, "I had practically nothing to eat today." Remember that "memory is the greatest liar of all." When you make a little list, the record is solid and inescapable.

It's not uncommon for a fat lady to delude herself, "I don't have to worry about my weight any more, I bought a new girdle." Or for a man to buy clothing two sizes too large in order to feel that he's thin. Instead be tough on yourself like the determined matron who told her waiter, "If I order dessert, say, 'Nix, Fatso!'"

If you find yourself making alibis for stopping your dieting, reread the common excuses that I've noted in chapter 11. Hopefully the answers will prevent you from making such excuses for yourself and will start you and keep you dieting successfully.

14. GETTING THE MOST FROM LOW-CALORIE FOODS

Low-calorie foods developed in the past few years amount to a small revolution in food processing and a great boon for dieters. Many of these foods are wholesome, nutritious and sometimes just about as delicious as their high-calorie counterparts. More and more women are beginning to take advantage of such reducing aids while shopping in the supermarkets.

If you're not getting all their slimming benefits now, you should start at once to help fill out your menus with low-calorie versions of such foods as available already. A supermarket checker complained that some women are beginning to ask him to add up the calories of the foods they buy, along with the prices. He told one, "You figure out your own calories, ma'am. I can only tell you what the stuff costs!"

One big advantage of these "low-calorie foods" is that you can count the calories right on the package as you buy and as you use them. This saves you the trouble of figuring out the calories for yourself from a chart or from the personal knowledge that you soon gain through the Stay Slim Eating method. Another asset is that you can't fool yourself into thinking that you're eating fewer calories than you actually are. The printed numbers on the packages don't lie (if they do, the maker is in for big trouble from the Food and Drug Administration).

There are so many new, low-calorie packaged foods appearing every month that you can now find them mixed in with the general foods. It pays to look for them in every department instead of, as formerly, in the "Diet Foods Section." It's not unusual, for example, to find low-calorie salad dressings displayed on the same shelves as the regular salad dressings.

There's a considerable difference in the calorie savings in salad dressings alone. A pint of one brand of low-calorie mayonnaise (imitation mayonnaise) contains about 2,300 calories fewer than a pint of regular mayonnaise. In taste tests, most people couldn't tell which brand was the regular mayonnaise and which was the low-calorie type, in spite of the enormous difference in calories. Just as many "testers," who were sure that they did detect a superiority, actually preferred the low-calorie type as those who selected the regular.

IMPORTANT: DON'T SHOW THE "LOW-CALORIE" PACKAGE

It's vital to realize that these people "testing their taste" consider themselves gourmets, not just ordinary eaters. If their highly-developed palates couldn't tell the difference between those low-calorie and regular foods in many categories (true in tests of carbonated beverages, also), it isn't likely that your family can either.

However, when people see the "low-calorie" label on the food before they taste it, then they're usually positive that the flavor is inferior. This too has been proved time after time. Therefore it's important that you don't show the "low-calorie" containers. Of course, if you're the cook, you can't fool yourself. However, you are certainly intelligent enough to decide the merit of a food on the basis of its actual taste rather than on prejudice against the flavor of low-calorie foods in general.

Even if the low-calorie food, in your naturally biased opinion, doesn't taste "quite as good" as the regular, isn't it worthwhile eating something not "quite as good" to help have a slim and attractive figure? Surely you can enjoy the dietary dressing which has only one to three calories per teaspoonful rather than ten times as many or more. This can make a big difference in preventing ugly pounds from piling on.

FLAVORS KEEP IMPROVING

It pays to keep trying the low-calorie foods even if you've been disappointed before in the past. Food processors are making great strides in improving flavors all the time. It wasn't until the time of this writing that I could find a low-calorie "mayonnaise" that I felt dieters would really enjoy. Those in the past had tasted flat or otherwise were unsatisfactory to the palate. So don't give up just because you were once disappointed. Keep on searching and tasting. It's worth it in order to help stay slim.

You can always get your money back from a reputable manufacturer by returning the product if you don't find it satisfactory. Don't hesitate to do this. For one thing, it's the quickest way for the maker to learn that he'd better improve his flavors or lose money in a hurry. By speaking up you help the food processor, other calorie-conscious people and yourself. What's more, you won't be wasting any money in case you can't use up the product.

Not so long ago the prices of low-calorie foods were much higher than the regular. In some cases, since the food processors were just beginning with such products, the costs of ingredients were higher. In others, the comparatively small amount produced, instead of great cost-reducing, production-line quantities, kept the prices high. Also, it's quite probable that in some instances, as one manufacturer admitted, "I charge more for low-calorie foods because I can get it."

Today the prices for both types are much more in line. The low-calorie "mayonnaise" mentioned was only a few cents more than the regular and can be ex-

pected to be about the same soon. As the demand for
the new type increases, savings can be effected by producing in larger quantities. Under our competitive system such savings will eventually be passed on to you.

Keep checking costs of regular versus low-calorie
foods at food markets; be wary of so-called "health
food stores" which usually get premium prices, way
out of line with reality. More and more you can find
comparable good values in canned fruits, vegetables,
jellies and many other popular foods. In some cases,
you'll learn that you can even save money. Non-fat
dry milk costs much less than regular whole milk, for
example. So does ice milk compared with ice cream in
many brands.

SOME OF THE BEST CALORIE-
SAVING FOODS

Non-fat instant dry milk has proved to be a great aid
to those who watch their weight. You get just as much
nutrition as with whole milk since only the butter fat
has been removed. But you save half the calories. The
flavor of non-fat dry milk has improved considerably
in recent years. It will probably become even better
in the future.

With this food, as with so many others (as covered
elsewhere), many people find that they prefer the
flavor of the low-calorie product after a while. I've
had many patients tell me that when they tried whole
milk later it made them feel a little ill as they found
the flavor and aftertaste "heavy and fatty."

The same was true with many individuals when
they switched from coffee and cream to black coffee
with or without artificial sweetening, when they eliminated use of butter or margarine as a spread or melted
on vegetables. (I have nothing against those fine foods
except for the excess of calories for weight-watchers.)

Most low-calorie beverages, as I've suggested often,
are just as tasty as those containing sugar but with

practically no calories at all. This development has been one of the greatest helps in reducing. A good, low-calorie carbonated drink is refreshing and satisfying. I often urge dieters to drink as many bottles a day as they wish. Such beverages satisfy the "sweet tooth," give a sense of filling the stomach temporarily, and are excellent "instead-of's" when you're about to reach for candy, cake, cookie or sugar-loaded, calorie-heavy beverage.

Always keep a plentiful supply of artificially sweetened sodas around in a variety of flavors, preferably in the refrigerator so you don't even have to go to the trouble of adding ice. You can drink a dozen different flavors in a day without adding a meaningful amount of calories to your day's consumption.

This applies not only to your stay slim eating habits, but also with any quick weight loss diet you use. These drinks have been lifesavers for many of my patients in helping to keep them from breaking a diet for want of a sweet soda, a malted, a confection, a cookie or another calorie-rich snack.

Hot and iced coffee (except where one or the other is forbidden on a few special situation diets) may be enjoyed as much and as often as you wish. Artificial sweeteners have made these drinks palatable for many who require the sweet taste in a drink. A refreshing glass of iced tea with a squeeze of fresh lemon and with artificial sweetening to taste, is every bit as delicious as "the real thing," without adding any calories which mount up to pounds of overweight.

Most fruit juices are now, or soon will be, available in lower-calorie, sugar-free form. These include apple, apple-grapefruit, apricot, orange, pineapple, pineapple-grape and many other combinations which satisfy and are usually enriched with added vitamins too. Keep in mind, however, that you are adding calories when you imbibe such fruit drinks, even though reduced considerably by the absence of added sugar. A typical 16-ounce can of artificially sweetened apple-grape juice is 80 calories total, 20 calories per 4-ounce serving. A 16-ounce bottle or can of artificially sweetened grape soda adds *no* calories to your intake.

Remarkable progress has been made in the artificial sweeteners themselves. You can get them and enjoy them in any form now—tablets, liquid, or crystals which are used by the spoonful like sugar. The old prejudice against sweetening with tablets or liquid instead of with crystals like sugar must necessarily be put aside as an alibi.

As for their safety as a food, thorough investigations to date haven't disclosed any findings that artificial sweeteners are unsafe for young or old. Like my Quick Weight Loss Diet, this advance makes it easier than ever before possible for you to slim down to your ideal weight and stay that way.

Many low-calorie "full course" meals are now on the market, with total calories marked on the package. If you don't find them fully satisfactory to the taste now, you may be sure that they will keep improving as the demand increases, as it inevitably must with more and more people realizing the essential health benefits of ideal weight. Furthermore, isn't it worth sacrificing a little "gourmet flavor" in some foods in order to look better, feel better and add years to your life?

You'll find such varied foods as chicken cacciatore, beef stew, chicken a la king and many other appealing specialties in low-calorie varieties at food markets. There are many types to choose from, including 300-calorie "full-course dinners" combining soup, a main dish and dessert—each in separate packets within one package.

Comparatively new are excellent selections of tuna fish, salmon, sardines and other fish with no oil added. These are especially delicious, with no oily taste, when prepared with a little imagination. Add fresh lemon juice, spices, herbs, ketchup, relishes, low-calorie salad dressings or mayonnaise substitutes. You'll enjoy thoroughly satisfying servings that reduce your calorie intake considerably compared with the "regular" servings.

The list of packaged "low-calorie" types of popular foods goes on and on including such favorites as:

Bread and crackers in low-calorie versions.

Sugar-free, high-protein cereals.

Artificially sweetened jellies, preserves and other fruit spreads.

Low-calorie pancake syrups.

Low-calorie cranberry sauce and other fruit sauces.

Artificially sweetened or no-sugar-added fruits and fruit cocktails. They're delicious and save many calories over fruits packed in the usual heavy, sugary syrups.

Salad dressings, touched on previously, now come in an infinite variety of low-calorie types—French, Italian, Thousand Island, Roquefort—you name it, you're likely to find it. You can also make your own low-calorie salad dressings using fresh lemon juice, vinegar, dry seasonings which come in envelopes, tomato juice and so on.

Desserts are available in many low-calorie forms. Artificially sweetened gelatin comes in many flavors, indistinguishable from the "real thing." There are low-calorie puddings, ice cream mixes, ice milk. Low-calorie whips from a package or pressurized can look like and substitute well for calorie-heavy whipped cream. And, of course, what is more refreshing for dessert than naturally low-calorie melon, with or without a touch of sherbet?

"From low-calorie soup to cheese" has now become a reality. Fat-free consommé and bouillon contain no calories to speak of. They may be enjoyed at meals and between meals instead of a snack loaded with calories. The hot or cold consommé will usually give you greater nutritional benefit too. There are various calorie-reduced cheeses including skim-milk cheeses, cheddar and cream cheese types, as well as delicious natural creamed cottage cheese, pot cheese and farmer cheese.

Artificially sweetened candy and chewing gum provide something sweet and satisfying when your appetite craves it, with very few calories added. Try the mints, candy drops and many other types such as gumdrops and hard candies. Candy mints and drops, only three calories each, now come in handy pocket rolls in many of the popular flavors, including chocolate, licorice, mint and fruit.

NEW FOOD-PROCESSING METHODS PRESERVE FLAVOR

If you were able to understand and know in detail the food-processing methods by which "low-calorie" foods are made, you'd realize that the quality can be as high and the products as "safe" and usually as nutritious as the higher-calorie processed foods. New techniques have been developed to take out much of the fat from meats by hand-trimming them first, then subjecting them to high-heat processing which removes the fat quickly and efficiently with a minimum of flavor loss.

Instead of oil in salad dressings, non-caloric vegetable colloids are used. Sauces are made with the aid of non-fat solids and low-calorie vegetable extenders instead of creams, starches and other high-calorie ingredients. High-calorie sugars are replaced by non-caloric sweeteners in making many dessert-type foods.

Natural shortcuts are used whenever possible, most of them being just good sense and ingenuity. In making low-calorie chicken dishes, for example, often only the white meat is used instead of dark meat which is higher in calories. The fatty skin is removed first.

New kinds of equipment have been devised. For making low-calorie soups and salad dressings, large, high-speed centrifuges are utilized. They whirl the fat to the surface. There it is quickly and thoroughly removed by special cooling and separation methods.

To add extra taste which may have been lost in the removal of fats, carefully selected extra-tasty vegetables, herbs and flavorings are used (more than may be common in high-calorie processed foods). Favorite ingredients include onions, garlic, spices, herbs and Italian tomatoes, all low in calories but high in the flavors that often distinguish gourmet foods. Wines and wine flavorings are used judiciously in order to add fine aroma and taste without many extra calories. All these excellent devices, long used by the "best cooks in town," help add delicious taste but very few calories.

In dressings, non-nutritive vegetable stabilizers are used frequently in place of heavy-calorie oils. That's why an ounce of low-calorie dressing may be only 15 calories compared with up to 150 calories per ounce of a similar "regular" dressing. Certainly that's a worthwhile saving when there's no vital loss of flavor.

Non-fat milk solids, a fine nutritive ingredient, are used as tasteful substitutes in many recipes, again bringing down the calorie totals considerably.

In lots of cases, although the price may necessarily be somewhat higher, the low-calorie product can taste better than the "regular" item. This is true, for example, with some preserves. A top-quality, low-calorie preserve on the market is made with 80 percent natural fruits, plus non-caloric sweeteners. Many "regular" preserves average about 45 percent fruit and 55 percent high-calorie sugar or other stretchers. Wouldn't you rather enjoy the low-calorie, almost-100-percent-fruit preserves as you get the benefits of fewer calories?

Even peanuts and other nuts which are normally very high-calorie are coming down in fat content. Using an oil-removing process developed by the U.S. Department of Agriculture, the nut retains much of its usual appearance without the smooth, oily look. Many people prefer the "dry-roasted" type of nut for flavor even without realizing that there is a reduction in calorie content.

However, you must still be careful not to eat even the dry-roasted type by the handful or you'll be adding a load of calories to your daily total consumption. The guideline must always be that if you do indulge in a high-calorie food occasionally (never when you're on the Quick Weight Loss Diet), the amount should be limited carefully.

As one case history of how helpful low-calorie foods can be, here are the results of a test conducted at a hospital under careful supervision. Fifty overweight men and women were told to eat the same quantities as they had in the past (not more) but substituting low-calorie foods for the regular foods.

At the end of a month, the average weight loss was 14 pounds. The doctor in charge of the test said that there were very few complaints about the quality and flavor of the low-calorie foods. He noted that the patients were well pleased with their meals, and especially with the drop in weight.

IMPORTANT WARNING ON LOW-CALORIE FOODS

While lots of the new foods save you many calories, you still must keep counting calories when eating them or your daily intake can go above the point where you take off weight. For example, a patient told me virtuously that she couldn't understand why she was gaining weight again after taking off many pounds on the Quick Weight Loss Diet. She said that on her Stay Slim Eating plan she was eating a number of "low-calorie" foods.

Upon questioning, I learned that she was eating loads of low-calorie foods *without counting the total calories*. For example, at lunch she'd have a whole 13¼ ounce can of low-calorie chicken a la king. When she brought in a duplicate can at my request, I showed her that the instructions suggested "three-ounce servings of 72 calories total." By eating the whole can at a meal, she was absorbing 324 calories. When she added vegetables and other foods, including too much "low-calorie pudding" on top of this, she was going way above her Stay Slim Eating allowance.

She learned her lesson, one that you must keep in mind for the rest of your life. She went back on the Quick Weight Loss Diet for a week which brought her down to her ideal weight again. She returned to Stay Slim Eating, using low-calorie foods sensibly. She has had little difficulty in maintaining her attractive slimmed-down figure since then.

Just because a package is labeled "low-calorie," "lower in calories," "sugar-free," "artificially sweetened" or some other such phrasing, gives you no license to eat limitless quantities. If you're not always careful you won't stay slim. Check the exact measurement in calories printed on the package.

Don't be fooled by "calories per three-ounce portion," for example, if such a portion of the food amounts to practically nothing in bulk and is not in fact even a moderate portion. Go by the *total calorie intake* involved. That's the only sure way to measure the number of calories you're adding at each meal.

COUNT CALORIES IN PREPARING SERVINGS

Your own intelligence and creativity can save many calories for yourself and your family in the preparation of foods. For example, you'll find that many recipes which call for whole milk can be made with skim milk and are just as delicious—some people say they're

even better. You can mix up as much skim milk as you
need at the time, using non-fat instant dry milk. That
saves you from keeping a bottle of milk handy and perhaps wasting money when it goes sour. More important, the skim milk cuts out half the calories compared with whole milk in the recipe.

You can keep finding more calorie-saving cooking
tips all the time in women's magazines and recipe
books. For example, if you like sour cream, which is
as high in calories as sweet cream, here's how you
can make a delicious substitute. Whip some creamed
cottage cheese in a blender to a smooth, sour-creamy
consistency. It's satisfying but with only a fraction
of the original calorie count.

To prove that a gourmet meal need not be high
in calories, consider this dinner menu:

Consommé with herbs, hot or jellied
Half a Cornish-rock hen, roasted in its own juices
   to a golden brown (no butter or margarine
   needed)
Asparagus with low-calorie "Hollandaise"
Endive salad with low-calorie Roquefort dressing
Minted melon balls, iced
Espresso coffee with artificial sweetener

For your own pleasant surprise, total up the calories
according to the earlier calorie listings for this fine
dinner. You'll see that this becomes a low-calorie meal
for your Stay Slim Eating. Here are just a few recipes,
chosen from many by food experts, to prove to you
that low-calorie servings can be delicious too:

Broiled half-grapefruit with mint garnish—75 calories
Melon-Balls-and-Strawberries, soaked in their natural juices and chilled thoroughly—half cup—55
   calories
Chilled Casaba Melon, moderate-sized wedge, garnished lightly with artificially sweetened mint
   jelly—80 calories

Broiled Banana, first lightly spread with artificially sweetened strawberry jelly—medium size—90 calories

Sherried Orange Sections, one orange sectioned, lightly soaked in sweet sherry and iced—40 calories

Eggs Arabesque, omelet of one egg, half tomato, ⅓ green pepper, herbs and spices—110 calories

Chicken Livers en brochette, 3 livers, 1 slice bacon, 4 mushroom caps—165 calories

Majorcan Fish Casserole, 1 slice red snapper, moderate portion rice, tomatoes, green pepper, saffron, in white wine—220 calories

Chinese Delight Omelet, 1 egg, 1 teaspoon each of mushrooms, celery, onions, green peppers, in no-fat fry pan—100 calories

Chicken Divan, 3 slices breast of chicken, ⅓ cup broccoli seasoned with herbs, 1 tablespoon Parmesan cheese—230 calories

Stuffed Baked Potato, small size, stuffed with 3 tablespoons of cottage cheese mixed and garnished with chives—90 calories

Ginger-Baked Carrots, 3 small carrots sprinkled with ginger and baked until tender—50 calories

Bibb-Artichoke Salad, sizable portion Bibb lettuce and 3 artichoke hearts, sprinkled with fresh lemon juice—50 calories

Asparagus Salad, 4 spears of asparagus, green pepper ring, low-calorie French or Italian dressing—85 calories

Orange-Ambrosia Cup, half fresh orange sectioned, soaked in light brandy, chilled on ice—75 calories

Orange-Grapefruit Royale, to fill medium-size dessert glass, mix orange and grapefruit sections with small cubes of artificially sweetened gelatine, garnished with small orange slice—45 calories

Springtime Fruit Cup, fill medium-size dessert glass with sliced fresh strawberries, diced fresh pineapple, fresh grapefruit sections, soaked in artificially sweetened lemon juice, garnished with mint leaf—45 calories

ZERO-CALORIE SERVINGS

Here are a few varied servings which show that some delicious foods can be eaten without consuming enough calories to even count them, such as:

Russian Borscht, dissolve 4 bouillon cubes in 4 cups of boiling water, cook with half-cup grated raw beets in covered saucepan 15 minutes, cool and chill, add 2 tablespoons of lemon juice just before serving, salt and pepper to taste, garnish with cucumber slice

Tomato-Celery Soup, dissolve 2 bouillon cubes in 2 cups of boiling water, in medium-size saucepan with 1 cup of finely diced celery, ¼ cup finely chopped onion, 1 cup tomato juice, salt and pepper to taste, simmer until vegetables are tender, serve hot

Mint Sauce, combine 2 tablespoons water, ½ cup vinegar, ½ teaspoon liquid no-calorie sweetener, leaves from 1 dozen sprigs of fresh mint finely chopped, let stand in warm place for about an hour

Cranberry-Orange Relish, put through food chopper with coarse plate 1 cup washed fresh cranberries and ½ unpeeled orange with seeds removed, stir in well 1 teaspoon no-calorie sweetener

These recipes are just a few of hundreds you can make with or without processed low-calorie foods to serve tasteful and satisfying low-calorie meals. Just a little extra care, and an attitude that Stay Slim Eating can also be enjoyable eating, can help keep health high and figures trim for you and your entire family.

If you become careless and the pounds start creep-

ing up on you once more, be sure to go back on the
Quick Weight Loss Diet or your choice of the other
quick reducing diets.

15. VITAL REDUCING ADVICE

Here is additional important and helpful information on some vital subjects only touched on previously.

DIETING FOR TEEN-AGERS AND CHILDREN

This book is written specifically to help overweight adults. The recommendations are therefore not necessarily for teen-agers and younger children, though I have helped hundreds of youngsters over a wide age range to reduce. I consider overweight at any age either immediately or potentially dangerous.

Unfortunately overweight parents are usually responsible for their children being fat. Studies show that when one parent is overweight, there is up to a 50% chance that the child will be too—and up to an 80% chance if both parents are heavies. When a mother and father are grossly overweight and try to get the child to reduce, it's little wonder that chances for success are small.

Children are primarily realists who believe, "Don't just tell me, show me." If you don't lose weight, there's far less chance that your child will, although some youngsters, especially when in their teens, exhibit more willpower than their parents.

Being overweight should not be considered a minor problem for a child. Surveys have shown that overweight children are generally more dependent to an undesirable degree. They have more school and sex problems, and are more often emotionally disturbed than youngsters of normal weight.

Despite old-fashioned ideas to the contrary, the fat child is not usually a healthier one. A leading pediatrician stated, "We don't want babies to be fat any more." If your child is overweight I urge you to discuss it thoroughly with your physician. Don't adopt the too-common attitude, "He (or she) will grow out of it."

Your doctor will determine whether or not your child is one of the tiny minority (usually noted as less than 5% or 1 out of 20) whose overweight is caused by some metabolic, glandular or other disturbance. Too often the fat child becomes a fat adult with all the great dangers involved.

Keep in mind that serious disorders adversely affected by overweight—including high blood pressure, diabetes and hardening of the arteries—may be started in the teens and perhaps even younger. There's no doubt that the spurt of growth during adolescence increases the body's nutritional needs, but when excess fat piles up that's a danger signal not to be ignored or misinterpreted as "nutritional need."

In dieting, children and teen-agers should be watched more closely for vitamin/mineral deficiencies although these are not likely to occur. The youngsters who are growing need more protein, calcium and iron than most adults, but properly planned food restrictions and increased exercise are often essential. Overweights, young or older, are usually less active, more sedentary and lethargic.

In a conference at the New York Academy of Medicine, it was stated that 15% of high school students are overweight (that's based on 10% or more over average weight). In cases where both parents were heavies, so were 73% of their offspring in this report. If you are a similar "case," I urge you strongly to do something at once to bring down your child's weight and your own. When both diet together, there's a better chance for both to succeed.

DIETING FOR ELDERLY PERSONS

Younger people can generally look to the elderly as good examples of losing weight rapidly when necessary, proving that it can be done. In my experience, when elderly persons are told to reduce because of coronary heart disease, peripheral vascular disease, generalized hardening of the arteries or for other reasons, they have little trouble staying on strict reducing diets. (If they had reduced earlier in life, most of them would not be afflicted so seriously now.)

These people know that this is their last chance to save themselves. The desire to live is strong in them and provides powerful motivation. They don't have to think about what may happen to them in 20 or 30 years, the problems and challenge are here and now. They will usually follow most any necessary regimen. They rarely break training when placed on a diet.

It has been recommended by the American Heart Association's Nutrition Committee that overweight can be prevented by cutting food consumption 1% every year after the age of 25. Instead of growing heavier as one grows older, as is common, the opposite should be true for better health and longer life. The elderly are generally less active and therefore not only should, but must, eat less if they wish to survive the menace to health brought on by forcing the heart to push around excess poundage.

Most individuals should remain at the same weight that they were in their upper teens (unless, of course, they were overweight then). Physiologically after those years the normal metabolism of energy usage by the body remains stationary. The amount of calories or energy necessary to sustain life and health decreases. But as individuals grow older and more prosperous they tend to eat more and get about less. Between the food intake increasing and the energy expenditure decreasing, an imbalance usually develops which piles up the calories on the plus side. The difference per day or week or month may be slight but as time goes on, the pound or 2 or 5 add up and total 20 to 50 or more extra pounds deposited over the years. This insidious slow deposit is the cause of most overweight.

Unfortunately these same persons cannot take off the weight gradually. They usually fail if they try. The elderly man or woman in imminent trouble because of excess fat cannot afford to wait for slow, gradual reducing even if it could work for them. Stringent dieting techniques, preferably under the care of a physician, will reduce the elderly patient as well as others swiftly, as required.

ADVICE ON EATING WHEN TRAVELING

The advice here primarily concerns eating while traveling outside the United States. Many patients who visit foreign countries return home either heavier, often to a considerable extent, or sick. It's vital in trying to avoid sickness of the stomach to understand the usual reasons why this occurs.

In general the European diet, as well as that in many other parts of the world, is given to an abundance of rich gravies, sauces and concoctions which mask the taste, and perhaps the toughness in the case of meats, of the original foods. Too often the fats or butter used in these sauces have been exposed for hours in a warmth where bacteria multiply very rapidly.

Such bacteria are often accidentally introduced into foods by careless cooks and handlers. It is a common practice in many places for the cook to taste the food frequently with a spoon or other utensil. This is reinserted without washing into the same mixture, perhaps time after time, communicating harmful bacteria if existent in that person.

Meanwhile, with the same general careless attitude, bacteria from a cold or sore throat shower the food via coughing and sneezing. This is less likely to happen in the "better" restaurants and hotels, but it is the desire and privilege of the traveler to seek out smaller and perhaps less careful eating places.

Good refrigeration which helps protect food from contamination is less likely to be found outside of the "best" hotels and restaurants. When foods cooked in heavy fats are eaten they are apt to upset the stomach, as would happen to the traveler who would eat too much fat at one time at home. Fats may often be overheated; this produces products of decomposition and often the result is indigestion, sometimes very severe.

Furthermore, travelers going abroad must be cautioned not to indulge heavily in foods to which they are unaccustomed. Spices, herbs and condiments are apt to be used more extensively. These tantalizing cooking tricks are employed to whet the appetite. People on holiday, tasting the enticing foods, usually eat far more than the body requires or can handle comfortably.

The result very frequently is painful and uncomfortable gastritis. If a few alcoholic drinks are added— cocktails plus wines or beer—there is an even greater chance of further inflaming the irritated, oppressed stomach.

It must be taken into account when traveling that rich, creamy foods such as custards and pastry fillings, especially when not properly refrigerated, are real culture media for staphylococcus germs. Food of this nature, particularly if exposed unrefrigerated for a few hours, not only encourages the germs to multiply rapidly but may produce enterotoxin which is very irritating for the gastric mucosa.

All travelers, especially those who are overweight,

are cautioned to observe the following basic rules as much as possible to avoid stomach upsets which may take severe and even serious forms:

1. Try very hard not to overstuff at any time. This gorging tends to aggravate the slightest undesirable condition that may exist. No matter how delicious a serving may be, it can be savored in a small or reasonable quantity instead of a huge overloading.

2. Drink only bottled water in most places.

3. Try to omit all rich gravies and sauces, heavy dressings and mayonnaise.

4. In most places it is much safer to bypass custards and rich, creamy pastries.

5. Though it may be difficult, try to be sure that the water for tea and coffee has really been boiled. This is particularly essential when ordering iced tea or coffee.

6. Avoid cold soups in many places, particularly cold creamed soups.

7. Be wary of any soft, cold concoctions.

8. Rare and medium rare foods in many places are dangerous, more so than well done foods.

9. Eat only when hungry—don't stuff a meal into yourself just because it's "mealtime." Such overstuffing can trigger upsets which might not have occurred otherwise.

10. In eating fruits and raw vegetables make sure, if possible, that they are thoroughly washed. It is better to avoid them.

11. In choosing from a menu it is generally safer to seek out those foods which are well boiled, baked or broiled.

12. If you feel ill, it can be very helpful to be carrying packets of instant oatmeal, bouillon cubes, whatever non-fatty, bland foods you can make just by adding *boiling* water.

It is difficult and perhaps at times impossible to diet, or to want to, when traveling—especially on vacation. The following menu is given as a relatively "safe"

day's eating, particularly if you are starting to feel
at all queasy or uncertain or if your stomach has given
any symptoms of upset:

Breakfast:
grapefruit or melon
1 hard boiled egg
1 slice of toast
hot coffee or tea (was the water boiled?)

Lunch:
clean, well-washed, tossed salad with vinegar and
a little oil only as dressing, or squeezed lemon
1 slice of toast
1 portion of cheese
black coffee or tea or bottled water

Dinner:
broiled steak, well done
well-washed sliced tomato
1 piece of well-washed fruit
black coffee or tea

With this type of eating you may not enjoy yourself
as much as some of the lucky ones who are not badly
affected. You will come back without dysentery, ty-
phoid brucellosis, amebic dysentery, salmonellosis or
attacks of acute indigestion. You will also return without having gained any weight or perhaps you will
even have lost a few pounds. At the very least, *keep
all the precautions in mind.* Bon voyage!

SMOKING AND OVERWEIGHT

Doctors all over the United States hear statements
like this from patients every day:

"Okay, Doctor, I'm finally scared enough of getting
lung cancer from smoking cigarettes that I want to
quit. But last time I tried, I gained 15 pounds in no

time even though I was already overweight. And I'm just as afraid of killing myself from being too fat. How can I stop smoking without putting on weight?"

When cigarette smoking is stopped, weight usually goes up. Yet it's possible to keep your weight down even when you stop smoking.

One man told me, "My doctor says he'll give me another month to take off the 18 pounds I put on since I stopped smoking, or else he'll put me back on cigarettes. He says that if it has to be one or the other with me, then overweight is more dangerous to my health than smoking."

That's true, as proved by facts and statistics. As you probably know from the U.S. Public Health Service Report: compared with non-smokers, average men smokers of cigarettes have about 10 times more chance of developing lung cancer. Heavy smokers are 20 times more likely to be stricken by lung cancer, along with other dangerous disorders. Smokers on an average die younger than non-smokers from many ills.

Overweight contributes to many disorders that are up to 15 times more serious than the possibility of getting lung cancer from smoking cigarettes. There's no question that you have a far better chance to live a longer, healthier and more vigorous lifetime if you slim down and don't smoke.

Here's why the smoker, man or woman, tends to put on weight when he stops smoking. He is usually a person who either by temperament or because he has so conditioned himself, seeks to satisfy every oral desire. As a smoker, he contents himself with cigarettes during his waking hours.

If he no longer has cigarettes, he usually seeks a substitute. He may take to eating candy, chewing gum, nibbling on fat-producing sweets and rich foods all day and evening. The pounds pile on and weight goes up shockingly.

A cigarette can be an appetite-curber in many ways. Some smokers find contentment in a cup of coffee and a cigarette. At coffee-breaks, the cigarette substitutes for a doughnut or pastry. At meals, many smokers take a cigarette instead of dessert. Some are happy with only a cigarette and coffee for breakfast. Thus a cigarette replaces some food hunger for them. But take away the cigarette and they tend to compensate for the loss of smoking habit and enjoyment by stuffing themselves with foods loaded with calories.

From a physiological or medical viewpoint, a cigarette may act as a weight-reducer in its effect on the system. This is true between meals but not with a cigarette smoked right after a meal, as explained later. Experiments have shown that nicotine works internally to reduce the extent that foods add to fat. When the smoker stops, the fat-inhibiting action halts too, usually accelerating weight gain.

Heavy smoking dulls, almost anesthetizes, the sense of taste. When smoking is stopped, foods taste better to the individual so that he or she is likely to eat far more and bigger portions, boosting the daily intake of calories considerably.

Here are specific steps to help keep you from gaining weight when you cut down on smoking or give it up completely:

1. Unless you're a supremely strong individual, it's practically impossible to go on a diet at the same time as you stop smoking cigarettes, and stick to either or both. In my practice the worst failures have been those patients who insisted on denying themselves both the foods and cigarettes they enjoyed so much, all at one time.

If you're overweight to start, go on the Quick Loss Diet at once to get down to your desired weight in a hurry. Meanwhile try to cut down on your smoking gradually over a period of weeks while you return to ideal weight. At that point you'll be better able to reduce smoking drastically or stop completely.

I've let my patients who are reducing smoke up to 10 cigarettes a day, except those who must stop all smoking immediately because of specific physical impairment. You can have a cigarette before meals as this tends to curb the appetite, and as you wish between meals, trying to space out your daily limit to 10 or preferably 6.

Don't inhale and don't take more than 10 easy puffs per cigarette. Then put out the cigarette and discard it or even keep it in your mouth unlit if you find that helpful. Filter cigarettes are preferable to all-tobacco, they usually contain less nicotine and other substances referred to as "tars." Choose filter cigarettes lowest in nicotine and tars. I consider them less harmful even though this may not have been clearly established statistically.

2. *Very important: Don't smoke a cigarette directly after a meal.* It's a curious fact that while a cigarette before a meal or between meals acts to burn up more fats and stimulates the metabolism, something quite the opposite happens directly after a meal. A cigarette in the middle or at the close of a meal induces a greater absorption of fat from the intestinal tract, tending to add more weight to your body.

If you "must" smoke, wait an hour or two after a meal before lighting a cigarette. If you can't do without a cigarette after the meal, take 3 or 4 slow, easy puffs, not inhaling, then put out the cigarette, holding it in your hand or mouth unlit if that's helpful.

3. If, like a small percentage of smokers and eaters who cut down, you experience "withdrawal symptoms," don't be frightened by them as possible deep-rooted physical ills. Such persons may develop some giddiness, exhaustion, headaches, drowsiness, restlessness, insomnia and a general feeling of uneasiness. An examination by your doctor is the best way to assure yourself that these are expressions of emotional conflict and not physical ills. He may prescribe tranquilizers or other measures.

Until you see your doctor, you may take available antihistaminics, "sleeping pills" which have been passed for non-prescription sale, 2 buffered aspirin tablets 4 times daily, common fizz alkalizers or just warm skim milk to help calm you.

4. After your weight is normal or near-normal, act to cut out smoking completely. It's not easy for most, so try every possible aid like the following to find what will work for you, trying one after the other or combinations if necessary.

Your doctor can help you with means such as injections of nicotine or nicotine-like substances to decrease or modify the craving for tobacco. He can prescribe tranquilizers and appetite-suppressing drugs or other medications such as astringent mouthwashes. In difficult cases the doctor should be seen at least weekly for his moral as well as medical support.

If you find it impossible to stop smoking completely, cut drastically to a "maintenance cigarette diet" of 6 cigarettes a day as there is little likelihood that this will be harmful. You might try switching to little cigars (as even some women are doing), regular cigars or a pipe. You're less likely to inhale since the stronger smoke is more alkaline and more irritating to the throat. Most cigar and pipe smokers tend to avoid the harsh irritation caused quickly by inhaling. (Inhaling cigar or pipe tobacco smoke is at least as bad for you as cigarettes.)

If you feel depressed as you quit smoking, drink strong coffee, tea or non-caloric carbonated beverages more often than usual, for a lift that has proved helpful for some people, without adding calories. You may be aided considerably by use of readily available anti-smoking tablets, lozenges, medicated chewing gum or other products, some of which contain a nicotine-like substance. Some people are helped by drawing on "smokeless cigarettes" made of plastic or other materials.

Try one after another of these suggestions until you find the one or combination that will help you stop smoking. It may be a tough fight but if you can cut out smoking cigarettes for 2 full days, usually the desire for another cigarette starts to diminish and then continues to lessen each day you abstain. The bright day finally comes when you can recall smugly, "Once I was a heavy smoker . . ."

After you take off the undesirable extra poundage quickly by the Quick Loss method, maintain your ideal weight as explained previously. You'll be much healthier for having overcome the dual dangerous problems of smoking and overweight.

CHOLESTEROL AND POLYUNSATURATES IN REDUCING DIETS

As knowledge has increased in the study of fats, involving the concentration of public attention on the potent words "cholesterol" and "polyunsaturates," the problem has become more rather than less complex for the experts, let alone for you.

Cholesterol is an essential fatty material which exists to some extent in the blood. It is not a fat in itself but is found associated with true fats in the animal body. The relationship between the availability of cholesterol and the mobilization of fats in body depots is an important one.

Too much cholesterol is bad for you; so is too little. If your doctor finds that you have a high blood cholesterol, he will restrict certain foods and recommend others for your case.

Since there is so much not determined definitely on the subject of cholesterol and polyunsaturates at this writing, certainly you cannot know how much each food affects you according to its cholesterol content. It is not even clear scientifically how much of the cholesterol in a food is absorbed by the body.

Your prime concern should not be the cholesterol content of foods or the lack or abundance of polyunsaturates, but rather following effective dieting procedures as recommended here. You'll be healthier when you're rid of excess fat, whatever causes it.

To clarify some terms: Saturated fats come from animal products chiefly (butter, lard, suet, certain oils), usually solidify at room temperature or lower, and tend to raise cholesterol levels. Unsaturated fats come principally from vegetable fats and are usually liquid at room temperature. Polyunsaturated fats have more hydrogens missing than usual unsaturated fats and they are more active in reducing blood cholesterol (many vegetable oils are high in polyunsaturates, but this is not true of coconut oil, olive oil or cocoa fat).

There seems little question that an elevated blood cholesterol level indicates that a person is more likely to have a heart attack than if he had a lower cholesterol level. It has not been proved conclusively that lowering the higher cholesterol level will specifically prevent heart disease, although indications point that way. Meanwhile I advise overweights as a whole to abstain from or reduce their intake of animal fats and high-fat dairy products in general.

In essence, I urge you to take steps now to get rid of your excess weight, while you let the scientists work out the facts in their area. The one point all agree on is that *overweights should reduce*.

SHOULD DRUGS BE USED IN DIETING?

Used correctly under the supervision of a physician only, drugs can be an excellent aid in reducing. So-called "reducing drugs" (often just vitamins) sold over the counter without a doctor's prescription, or not specifically designated for you by a physician, should never be taken for dieting. Drugs are seldom required for the person who has a compelling and driving desire to reduce. Some individuals need every means available to assist them in their reducing. For them the physician has many good drugs to choose from for various purposes. He alone knows when to give drugs, when to increase or diminish dosage, when to stop their use. The giving of drugs is a very intimate and skillful art. It cannot be delegated to the lay person, nurse, dietician or druggist.

I have prescribed drugs for patients, including some of the cases cited in this book, with fine effect. I've always checked usage closely and have had only benefits, no harmful results. I deplore the attitude of too many professionals and others who say flatly, "The use of drugs in reducing is bad"—usually because of cases of improper usage. That's like saying, "The use of autos is bad and should be abolished," because some people drive improperly and accidents occur.

Of the many drugs helpful in reducing I've found the appetite depressants and suppressants most valuable. (Technically, for the curious, most reducing drugs may be classified under anorectics, belladonna preparations, diuretics, hormones, intestinal bulk producers, sedatives and tranquilizers, and various combinations.) In my experience, drugs I've prescribed as reducing aids are not habit-forming for 99% of the patients using them. Many who start with them drop their use as soon as they become accustomed to the dieting regulations.

Drugs are useful in reducing the appetite, counteracting mental depression and physical lethargy, increasing mental interest and physical activity, ridding the body of excess salts and liquid and many other functions.

Leave the knowledge and responsibility of drug usage to your physician. Don't worry about relationship to strange terms you may have come across in respect to reducing, such as "appestat . . . thermostat . . . automatic appetite control centers" in the brain or elsewhere in the body. Such words usually serve only to confuse.

Your job is to follow all dieting instructions explicitly, especially when taking drugs. Don't juggle your medicines as suits your fancy. Don't increase or decrease dosage on your own. If you experience worrisome symptoms, inform your physician at once.

Concentrate on your dieting and on continuing to lose dangerous excess weight. Don't become upset by your own fears or any admonitions from others if your physician prescribes drugs as reducing aids. As stated in the Journal of the American Medical Association, "Drugs have a decided role in the treatment of obesity, especially in the first 4 to 8 weeks."

"SEE YOUR DOCTOR?"

Of course, as advised on other pages, it's best to see your doctor before and during dieting. He will check your physical condition thoroughly and inform you accordingly, including use of drugs or not. My recommendations here are for people without serious disorders such as diabetes, hyperthyroid, Addison's disease, gastric or intestinal ulcers, cirrhosis of the liver, malignancy, tuberculosis, ulcerative colitis or neurotics for whom dieting creates added problems. Persons with any such disorders should go on a reducing diet only under the close and constant supervision of a qualified physician. And whether on my diets or any others, if you feel any severe, unusual symptoms at the start or at any time, stop the dieting procedure and see your doctor.

However I must emphasize this: It is more important for most of those with diabetes and other serious disorders to get down to the ideal weight and to stay slim than for others. Your doctor will confirm this.

In reality, few people with the serious medical disorders mentioned are fat. Before diabetics reach a serious stage, they may be heavy, then they are forced to reduce. The great majority are rarely overweight because the severe illnesses have already caused them to reduce either because of lack of appetite or on a doctor's deadly serious orders. It's significant too that overweights with such disorders have usually reduced on what are really quick action diets like mine, of the doctor's choosing.

If you're suffering from diabetes or another serious medical disorder and are overweight, you may be able to use diets in this book under your doctor's supervision, as has been done with many of my patients. I've had excellent results with diabetics on the Quick Weight Loss Diet, with gallbladder patients on a fat-free diet, with hypertensives on many disciplined diets which help reduce the blood pressure effectively.

We must be sensible about the advice to "see a doctor." Most overweights won't go to the doctor about reducing. They don't consider obesity the deadly sickness that it is. Actually if 23 million or more over-weights swarmed into doctors' offices, the physicians wouldn't have time to take care of other ills.

Medical journals have noted that if the usual advice were observed such as, "If you have a heavy cold, see a doctor"—then physicians could take care of little else. Americans average 4 to 5 colds a year. If only 1 a year was a heavy cold, this would mean some 185 million doctor visits for colds alone.

Preferably with your doctor's checkup, the prime objective for people without serious ailments must be to get those excess pounds off, not just for improved appearance but to prevent tragic afflictions due to overweight.

NO MIRACLES IN HEALTH FOODS AND FADS

Much dieting advice is doled out by the "nature boys," the "naturopathic advisers" and other such self-styled nutritionists, lecturers and "natural food" advisers. Most of these self-appointed experts insist that the inherent qualities of life, health and beauty can be found only in a return to the primitive in food, clothing, love or variations on that theme. Only the "natural foods" they recommend are supposed to be good for you, all deviations are bad.

If these people wish to delude themselves that wheat germ, blackstrap molasses, brewer's yeast, seaweed, licorice, yogurt, grapes and other hallowed items have special health-giving and beautifying qualities, that is their privilege. *You must realize, beyond question, that such foods have no greater quality for sustaining life than other natural, processed or concentrated foods have which are readily available and usually far less costly.*

Some of these advisers back the eating of only vegetables, or only fruits, or meats and salads and no other foods, or other systems. Many of the recommendations are excellent ways of reducing. They usually eliminate the rich calories in pies, pastry, ice cream and heavy dressings. One of the leaders who speaks and writes of "wonder foods and diets" fundamentally specifies a meal consisting of a salad, meat, some fruit as dessert, and black coffee. This comprises a fine reducing diet, no matter who advises it. There is no danger in this diet, as there is little likelihood of damage from the most lopsided diets if they are not extended over a long period of time.

The real danger is not so much that these "health foods" usually cost much more and thus in effect cheat you but that they undermine confidence in excellent staple foods. Far worse, the faulty preachings may keep people from seeing a physician for proper treatment of arthritis, cancer and other serious ills. The health foods are regarded as cure-alls by too many gullible people.

The statistics again are the best proof that a return to the "old-fashioned ways of eating and living" would be damaging and dangerous rather than helpful. In 1900 the average life expectancy was under 50 years of age; today it is 70 or over. The American Medical Association's Council on Food and Nutrition states,

"There are no *health* foods." The usual foods available in most food stores are healthful for the vast majority of persons when not overeaten to the point of piling up deposits of excess fat.

SEXUAL POTENCY AND OVERWEIGHT

"Does sexual potency increase as overweight diminishes?" I've been asked that question hundreds of times. The answer is necessarily unclear because so much of the relationship between sex and overweight depends on individual temperament and psychological factors.

I've had some male patients tell me that while they were reducing and after they lost a good deal of weight their sex desires and physical abilities had increased greatly. Women have told me the same about their husband's actions when slimmed down, along with their personal increased sexual desires. However these reports are not sufficient to provide an average or covering answer.

The sex act itself is not hampered by overweight unless layers of fat inhibit the organs and cause difficulties. The libido and passions are not necessarily disturbed by excess weight, although a general lethargy and lessening activity produced by overweight may affect sexual desires and capacities adversely.

One cannot overlook individual attitudes and cultural mores. Only 40 to 80 years ago, most of the "beautiful women" in America were 20 or more pounds overweight by today's standards. Currently the slim figure is commonly regarded as most attractive and appealing whereas the fat man or woman usually draws a sharply negative "Ugh!" from the opposite sex. Of course some cultures still glamorize the meaty mate as the most desirable sex symbol.

It is my belief that a relatively small increase in weight does not diminish the sexual drive on the average. But as overweight increases, greater fatigue is caused by the sexual act as by general exercises and activities which require physical exertion. Conversely, as the overweight takes off debilitating poundage, his general sense of well-being, vigor and energy usually increases.

It is a known fact among gynecologists that a reduction of weight is usually accompanied by increased fertility, but there is certainly no guarantee that this will be so in each case.

You may have read here and there that some overweight men and women are glad and even eager to be fat in order to escape the attentions of the opposite sex, marriage proposals and involvements. In my practice exactly the opposite has been true. One of the greatest motivations for reducing among my patients has been the desire by women to slim down in order to attract a man for marriage or to reattract a straying husband—or by men to be more appealing to women or to win back an increasingly indifferent wife.

Among the gratifying comments I've heard repeated many times by patients is a man's, "I feel like a new man!" and a woman's, "I feel like a bride again!" and, "They tell me I look years younger!" If such a result holds high promise for you and decisive motivation for reducing, make the most of it. I cannot promise the dieter greater sexual fulfillment but I can emphasize the incontrovertible statistics that point to more youthful appearance, better health, greater vigor and longer life when not fat.

EXERCISE AND WEIGHT LOSS

Proper exercise is a valuable asset to a reducing program. A special report by a committee of the American Medical Association stated that there is some evidence to suggest that exercise has a beneficial effect on metabolic functions that combat obesity, in addition to burning calories.

It's desirable to exercise all your life, modifying and slowing down the competitive forms as age progresses. Many exercises are fine at any age: walking, bicycling, gardening, dancing. Choose the form of exercising and sports that appeals most to you and go at it daily for long enough to do you good, but stop at the slightest hint of exhaustion.

When you walk, move briskly, purposefully. If you saunter lazily you won't be getting much exercise. Lift your chest, pull in your abdomen (tell yourself as you walk, "AbdomIN!") and stride alertly, conscious of the movements of your legs and body. Your muscle tone and posture will benefit.

A very simple exercise to help you flatten your stomach bulge is this. Pull in your abdomen as though you're trying to make it touch your spine, while you breathe naturally and count to yourself slowly to 10. Do this while standing and walking, at least a half dozen times a day. In a month or two your abdomen will be flatter and firmer. Also your posture will be improved.

Exercise is a highly recommended aid, but keep this in mind always: *no amount of exercising will reduce you if you overeat.* To get down to ideal weight, combine proper exercising with swift reducing on the Quick Weight Loss Diet.

APPROXIMATE CALORIES USED UP PER HOUR BY ACTIVITIES

To help you understand how many calories are used up by the body when you're active rather than inactive, note the listing that follows. The figures are necessarily approximated since each individual exercises, works or walks with differing energy usage. A 120-pound woman uses about 240 calories per hour when doing active housework such as using a vacuum

sweeper. She uses up only about 84 calories per hour
when sitting and resting, talking, reading, knitting, and
so on.

	120 *lb. woman*	160 *lb. man*	*per lb.*
Bicycling, moderate	192	256	1.6
Bicycling, energetic	480	640	4.0
Cooking, active	96	128	.8
Dancing, moderate	264	352	2.2
Dressing, undressing	96	128	.8
Driving auto	108	144	.9
Eating	84	112	.7
Exercise, moderate	240	320	2.0
Gardening, active	276	368	2.3
Golf	144	192	1.2
Housework, active	240	320	2.0
Ironing	120	160	1.0
Laundry, moderate	120	160	1.0
Lying at rest	60	80	.5
Office work, active	120	160	1.0
Painting furniture	144	192	1.2
Ping Pong	300	400	2.5
Piano Playing	132	176	1.1
Rowing	600	800	5.0
Running	444	592	3.7
Sawing wood	372	496	3.1
Sewing, knitting	84	112	.7
Sitting at rest	84	112	.7
Skating	252	336	2.1
Skiing	624	832	5.2
Standing	84	112	.7
Swimming	480	640	4.0
Tennis	336	448	2.8
Typing	108	144	.9
Walking moderately	168	224	1.4
Writing	84	112	.7

You'll realize from such figures that even walking at

moderate speed for a full hour, while excellent exercise for your body, uses only about 200 calories. So you still must watch your calorie *consumption* carefully. You can't let yourself go and eat a lot at the next meal just because you exercised for an hour or more.

EXERCISING TO HELP YOUR FIGURE

There are many different exercises which will help keep your figure trim all over and which can help to firm your abdomen and other parts of the body. Here are a few exercises you may wish to try as a start. To get the most good from any exercising you should do it continuously for 15 minutes or more and day after day. Proper exercising helps to tone up the system and improve the circulation, as well as aiding toward having a trim physique.

A few cautions are essential about exercising. If your legs tend to be thick and heavy, for example, don't expect any "miracle" transformations. Proper diet and exercise will help your legs to become as slim and trim as possible but cannot change the basic structure. The same applies to other parts of the body.

Never exercise to the point of exhaustion or feeling any pain. Don't overexert. If it hurts, stop—it's bad for you; continue later or the next day.

Try all or as many of the following exercises as you wish. Start by doing each or several of the exercises just a few times. Then increase the number of times you perform each exercise day after day.

To Help Trim Figure:

1. Stand erect. Holding arms straight in front, clasp your hands. Very slowly bring arms forward and overhead. In that position, roll head back as far as possible without straining, then roll head to the right, then to the left, then to the front. Slowly bring down

arms forward, hands still clasped, to original position. Repeat 10 times.

2. Stand erect, arms straight forward. Swing right leg slowly up forward, then far back, then bring to rest on floor as you were. Do the same with the left leg. Repeat five times alternately with each leg.

3. Stand erect, arms relaxed at sides. Bring left knee slowly up to your chest, bending upper torso and head forward, clasping leg to chest with hands. Return to original position. Do the same with the right leg. Repeat five times alternately with each leg.

4. Stand erect with hands on shoulders. Bend forward slowly as far as you can comfortably, holding upper torso straight. Then bend slowly from hips to right, then back, then to left, then forward, then back to original erect position. Now repeat the cycle, starting this time by bending forward, then to left, back, right, forward, up again. Repeat five times each alternating cycle.

To Help Slim Waist and Flatten Rear, Firming Legs and Thighs:

1. Stand upright with arms held straight up overhead. Bend forward from hips, letting upper body relax, head and arms hanging loose, not trying to touch the floor. Keeping relaxed, bend knees slightly, then holding arms forward return to original upright position, arms straight up. Repeat slowly 10 times.

2. Sit back in a straight, hard, armless chair, holding chair seat with both hands. Raise right leg, hold straight forward, move back and forth about 18 inches, repeat 10 times.

Lower right leg, raise left leg and repeat the same exercise 10 times with left leg.

Lean back, hold tight to chair seat, lift both legs together straight forward, then holding both legs tight together move them from side to side about 18 inches, repeat 10 times.

With both legs straight forward, move one leg after another up and down like scissors blades, 10 times.

In same position, holding legs straight forward, cross one over another alternately, 10 times.

3. Take kneeling position, spread legs apart slightly, thrust arms down between legs, and rest hands on the floor. Moving the knees, "bounce" your rear up and down slowly 10 times.

To Help Slim and Firm Legs, Also Abdomen:

1. Lie flat on back on floor, arms straight out at sides at right angles to torso. Bend right knee up. Keeping knee bent, turn leg to left, trying to touch floor with right knee at left side of body without straining. Return slowly to original position. Go through same action with left knee, trying to touch it to floor at right side of body, then bringing it back to original position. Repeat five times alternating with each leg.

2. Lie flat on back on floor, legs straight forward on floor, arms back over head resting on floor. Bend both knees together up close to stomach and clasp rather tightly, but without strain, with both hands. Return arms slowly overhead as you straighten both legs together up toward the ceiling, then lower them together, held straight, to the floor. Repeat slowly entire action 10 times.

To Help Slim Upper Arms:

1. Stand ĕrect, arms down at sides. Raise arms slowly upward by bringing straight out at each side until palms are flat against each other overhead. Now face palms outward and keep arms straight, return in sideward motion slowly to straight down. Repeat 10 times.

2. Stand erect, arms at sides. Raise arms straight overhead, palms facing each other and about 12 inches apart. Turn palms toward back wall. Make tight fists. Pull arms down slowly, bending elbows, as if pulling

weighted ropes down from ceiling, until fists are at shoulder height. With fists still clenched, raise arms slowly as if pushing weight up until arms are straight. Repeat up-down action slowly 10 times.

To Help Tighten Under-Chin: Sit well back in a hard, straight, armless chair. Let arms hang down loose at sides. Sit straight, shoulders back, but not tense. Move head as far back as you can; in that position open mouth wide, then close slowly. Open and close mouth slowly 10 times. Do at least three times daily. This also helps to relax you, as does all good, moderate exercising.

ACTIVITY HELPS MAINTAIN HEALTH AND SLIMNESS

No matter how inactive you may have been in the past, or in recent years, you'll find that you'll enjoy activity, exercise and sports very much once you make them a natural part of your living pattern. Instead of going everywhere by auto, try to make it a habit to walk to your destination if not too distant. Instead of sauntering along, walk briskly with shoulders back and head high. Take strides that require some energy and use up more calories than in strolling.

Instead of hopping into a car without thinking, to go to the store or mail a letter, walk if it's not more than 15 minutes or so away. Instead of sitting and chatting with a neighbor or friend, suggest that both of you talk while walking briskly. Instead of hailing a cab to take you to a restaurant not too far away, enjoy the benefits of walking there and back.

As for sports, you don't have to be an athlete to get lots of good from them. As you slim down from the Quick Weight Loss Diet or other effective diets, you'll find that you'll get a lift mentally as well as further health benefits from bicycling, swimming, walking and other physical activity.

Philosophically, too, you might consider the advice of Diogenes: "By constant exercise one develops freedom of movement—for virtuous deeds."

YOUR DECISION: EAT TO LIVE . . . OR . . . LIVE TO EAT

I am most hopeful that this book will lead you to take the necessary and effective steps to reduce—starting right now. I urge you, for your health's sake, to use these recommendations which I've developed during my own lifetime in medicine.

As I have done, along with many thousands of patients, use these suggestions to get down to your ideal weight, and then to maintain that reduced weight. The Quick Weight Loss Diet, Combination Plan with Stay Slim Eating and other procedures and tips which have helped so many thousands to reduce successfully can work for you too.

Many of my greatest satisfactions as a doctor have come from watching the obstinately and persistently overweight in my care—particularly those who had tried and failed for years to reduce—finally succeed through my methods. I wish you the same success and the same gratifying results—a more attractive body, greater freedom of movement, more vigorous and sustaining health, and a better chance for a longer, happier, more rewarding life.

*Biggest dictionary value
ever offered in paperback!*

The Dell paperback edition of

THE AMERICAN HERITAGE DICTIONARY
OF THE ENGLISH LANGUAGE

- Largest number of entries—55,000
- 832 pages—nearly 300 illustrations
- The only paperback dictionary with photographs

These special features make this new, modern dictionary clearly superior to any comparable paperback dictionary:

- More entries and more illustrations than any other paperback dictionary
- The first paperback dictionary with photographs
- Words defined in modern-day language that is clear and precise
- Over one hundred notes on usage with more factual information than any comparable paperback dictionary
- Unique appendix of Indo-European roots
- Authoritative definitions of new words from science and technology
- More than one hundred illustrative quotations from Shakespeare to Salinger, Spenser to Sontag
- Hundreds of geographic and biographical entries
- Pictures of all the Presidents of the United States
- Locator maps for all the countries of the world

A DELL BOOK 75c

If you cannot obtain copies of this title from your local bookseller, just send the price (plus 15c per copy for handling and postage) to Dell Books, Post Office Box 1000, Pinebrook, N. J. 07058. No postage or handling charge is required on any order of five or more books.

75¢

DELL
75¢
REF

Dell
0207

Based on the new best-selling
AMERICAN HERITAGE DICTIONARY—
the freshest, most innovative, most useful dictionary
to be published in this century

THE
AMERICAN HERITAGE
DICTIONARY
OF THE ENGLISH LANGUAGE

- Largest number of entries—55,000

- 832 pages—nearly 300 illustrations

- The only paperback dictionary with photographs

440-00207-075

DELL

AMERICAN HERITAGE
DICTIONARY

HOW MANY OF THESE DELL BESTSELLERS HAVE YOU READ?

Fiction

1. **THE NEW CENTURIONS** by Joseph Wambaugh $1.50
2. **THE TENTH MONTH** by Laura Z. Hobson $1.25
3. **THE SCARLATTI INHERITANCE** by Robert Ludlum $1.50
4. **BLUE DREAMS** by William Hanley $1.25
5. **SUMMER OF '42** by Herman Raucher $1.25
6. **SHE'LL NEVER GET OFF THE GROUND** by Robert J. Serling $1.25
7. **THE PLEASURES OF HELEN** by Lawrence Sanders $1.25
8. **THE MERRY MONTH OF MAY** by James Jones $1.25
9. **THE DEVIL'S LIEUTENANT** by M. Fagyas $1.25
10. **SLAUGHTERHOUSE-FIVE** by Kurt Vonnegut, Jr.   95c

Non-fiction

1. **THE SENSUOUS MAN** by "M" $1.50
2. **THE HAPPY HOOKER** by Xaviera Hollander $1.25
3. **THE GRANDEES** by Stephen Birmingham $1.50
4. **THE SENSUOUS WOMAN** by "J" $1.25
5. **I'M GLAD YOU DIDN'T TAKE IT PERSONALLY** by Jim Bouton $1.25
6. **THE DOCTOR'S QUICK WEIGHT LOSS DIET** by Irwin Maxwell Stillman, M.D. and Samm Sinclair Baker $1.25
7. **NICHOLAS AND ALEXANDRA** by Robert K. Massie $1.25
8. **THE GREAT AMERICAN FOOD HOAX** by Sidney Margolius $1.25
9. **THE DOCTOR'S QUICK INCHES-OFF DIET** by Stillman & Baker $1.25
10. **SURROGATE WIFE** by Valerie X. Scott as told to Herbert d'H. Lee $1.25